CW00434045

VAGUS NERVE

*How to Activate the Natural Healing Power of
Your Body with Self-Help Exercises and Techniques
to Reduce Inflammation, Chronic Illness, PTSD,
Trauma, Anxiety and Depression*

By John P. Atkinson

© Copyright 2019 By John P. Atkinson - All rights reserved.

This content is provided with the sole purpose of providing relevant information on a specific topic for which every reasonable effort has been made to ensure that it is both accurate and reasonable. Nevertheless, by purchasing this content, you consent to the fact that the author, as well as the publisher, are in no way experts on the topics contained herein, regardless of any claims as such that may be made within. As such, any suggestions or recommendations that are made within are done so purely for entertainment value. It is recommended that you always consult a professional prior to undertaking any of the advice or techniques discussed within.

This is a legally binding declaration that is considered both valid and fair by both the Committee of Publishers Association and the American Bar Association and should be considered as legally binding within the United States.

The reproduction, transmission, and duplication of any of the content found herein, including any specific or extended information will be done as an illegal act regardless of the end form the information ultimately takes. This includes copied versions of the work both physical, digital, and audio unless express consent of the Publisher is provided beforehand. Any additional rights reserved.

Furthermore, the information that can be found within the pages described forthwith shall be considered both accurate and truthful when it comes to the recounting of facts.

As such, any use, correct or incorrect, of the provided information will render the Publisher free of responsibility as to the actions taken outside of their direct purview. Regardless, there are zero scenarios where the original author or the Publisher can be deemed liable in any fashion for any damages or hardships that may result from any of the information discussed herein.

Additionally, the information in the following pages is intended only for informational purposes and should thus be thought of as universal. As befitting its nature, it is presented without assurance regarding its prolonged validity or interim quality. Trademarks that are mentioned are done without written consent and can in no way be considered an endorsement from the trademark holder.

Table of Contents

Introduction

Chronic stress overload increases the risk for a number of conditions that commonly affect many people. It is important to deal with stress and anxiety in the healthiest and most natural ways possible. The techniques in this book are all you need to enhance the quality of your life and beat stress and anxiety.

Anxiety and pain can take over your life if you let them. They can affect your health in a tremendous way. Therefore, taking actions to reduce your pain and anxiety is vital.

Don't panic, take a deep breath and relax; help is at hand if you are reading this book and you suffer from inflammation, chronic illness, PTSD, trauma, anxiety and depression. This book will help give you a practical, no-nonsense approach to dealing with the aforementioned disorders.

Each of these sections are designed to offer a different angle on how to activate your vagus nerve, from health and diet, to the simple natural healing power of your body with self-help exercises and techniques that anybody can learn and use.

There is no need to continue living with these disorders. You can put an end to them. Self-awareness is the key. In applying what you learn in this book you will equip yourself with remedies that are safe and easy to get.

By the time you're done with this e-book, you're going to feel **inspired**. You're going to want to run out and tackle any of the challenges that had been dogging you for so long. So, what are you waiting for? Let's find out how to cure your vagus nerve naturally, safely, and in a wonderfully healthy way so you can start living the stress-free life that you deserve.

Chapter 1: Understanding Anxiety, PTSD, Trauma and Depression

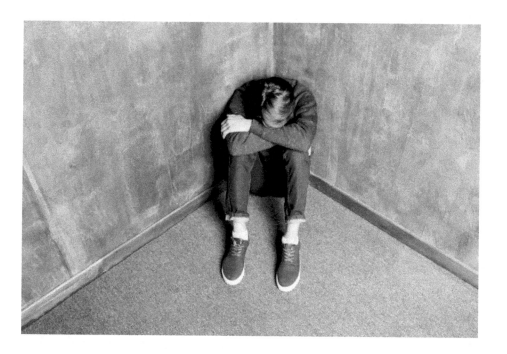

What is Stress?

Stress is a word that is often heard and talked about but truly, not fully understood. Some people consider stress as an event that happens in their lives, like losing a job or experiencing an accident or injury. Some people on the other hand would say that stress is the behavior of the body towards certain events such as nail biting or anxiety.

In actuality, stress involves both the event and response of the body and mind to the so-called stressor (source of stress). When a person undergoes a situation, it is automatically evaluated by the mind mentally. The mind decides if the situation is a threat then generates logic on how to deal with the situation at hand, and if the person has the skill to solve the problem. If it is decided that the skills acquired by the person is not enough to handle the problem, then the situation is labeled "stressful". If the situation is something the person can handle, then it is considered otherwise.

There are many sources of stress. Contrary to common belief, it is not always sourced from a negative situation. It could also be caused by positive situations like a job promotion or a new baby. The body experiences stress even in these positive changes, because it has to adapt to new challenges. For some people, being flooded with added work and activities could cause enormous stress. Another good example of a positive situation that can cause stress is pregnancy or giving birth. For a mother especially that is experiencing pregnancy for the first time, the body experiences enormous change. These changes may cause imbalances on the body, therefore releasing stress hormones. When the baby is born, both the father and mother will experience changes in their lifestyle if not properly conditioned for these changes. This situation also triggers stress.

Even if you don't struggle with anxiety and panic attacks on a daily basis, internalized stress can still silently wreak havoc on your body and mind, leaving you incredibly vulnerable to long-term health problems and causing you to underperform in aspects of your life. This is no way to be living. We need to treat mental health just as seriously as we would any illness, and need to do something now before it gets worse. But what can we do?

What is Anxiety?

Anxiety is a normal feeling but it is considered a disorder or problem once the symptoms interfere with an individual's ability to function normally.

Without feelings of anxiety, it's likely that our ancestors would not have survived very long or that the human race would have been so successful. For our ancestors, anxiety at the sight of a prowling lion sent adrenaline through their systems, which prompted the "fight or flight" response and helped them to live another day.

Today, anxiety remains a common emotion, but the focus is often shifted to more abstract, and usually more trivial issues, rather than prowling predators. Bill payments, worries over jobs, loss, or divorce all stimulate feelings of uncertainty and anxiety. Even relatively mundane things such as going out, being late, and tests can cause anxiety to flare up. The emotion becomes a disorder when we fail to control our worries and concerns; some people are able to do this more effectively than others. For those with normal anxiety responses the emotion is quickly dispelled, but for those with an anxiety disorder this is much harder and the condition can affect every aspect of their daily lives – in some cases to a crippling extent.

Anxiety is very bad for your health in many different ways, unfortunately it is often looked at as the enemy in our culture rather then something which can teach us something about ourselves. Therefore, the goal for most people is to get rid of it, usually with medication instead of understanding it and healing it naturally. It is vital that you take control over your life and conquer the anxiety you might have.

A person experiencing anxiety can certainly manage to cope enough to get through their day, but that anxiety is taking a toll on their life. It's building stress around them and it can increase the risk of some serious health conditions, including heart attacks, strokes, panic attacks, and much more.

What is PTSD or Post-Traumatic Stress Disorder?

Life is unpredictable, there are chances you have had some horrible physical or emotional traumas that have left a distressing mark on you. A loved one's death or a horrifying accident is an example. It is possible that just being witness to a situation can cause PTSD. Some of the symptoms include reliving the trauma, responding to a similar situation frantically, or always being apprehensive that it can occur again. You might feel detached or disinterested, far worse you might become emotionally numb if not attended to.

This can develop once someone has experienced or witnessed something very difficult, violent, or traumatic. They often relive something painful repeatedly, and might be withdrawn emotionally, get angry fast, or have outbursts. The symptoms of PTSD might start right away, or could come on years after the incident or incidents. Physical attacks, natural disasters, and war are all common triggers of PTSD, and anxious episodes can come on with no signs or warnings.

This condition is usually triggered by real events in life; these are usually serious and very frightening. They include involvement in road accidents, violent assault (including sexual assault), witnessing violent events, military combat, witnessing or being involved in terrorist attacks or severe natural disasters. Not everyone involved in traumatic events develops the condition, but estimates suggest that up to 30 % of those involved in traumatic situations will develop PTSD.

What is Depression?

Depression is caused by changes in life circumstances, grief, stress, alterations in hormone levels, medical conditions, and several other traumatic and overwhelming demands of life. These factors alter the brain chemistry. The onset of depression and its expression differs among people. How people deal with grief is in part influenced by their genetic patterns.

Depression is linked to the state of our heart, our heart is linked to our emotions or feelings, and our emotions or feelings are linked to our thoughts. If you feel overwhelmed or anxious about a situation or unforeseen circumstances have made a significant impact in your life, and you don't get the right psychological support or tools to help you, this can have a long-term effect on the state of your heart and mental health. Deferred hope and storing anxiety in our heart can weigh us down, causing us to experience depression. This is why the mental illness approach to depression can keep us stuck in a cycle of depression because it doesn't give us hope that we will ever be able to move forward and live a life free from depression. We need to take a new approach when providing therapy to people who suffer from depression, and that approach is giving them the strategies to improve their mental health which provides them with hope instead of teaching people they will always have a mental illness.

Often, we focus solely on our minds when it comes to depression. Yes, our minds are essential but our heart, emotions, and thoughts are all interrelated, and we must pay attention to all of these precious parts of our inner self and physical body. I completely respect the medical field and all the fantastic people who work in that industry. However, the medical field often treats our physical symptoms and diagnoses our situations based on what our physical body is telling us, but how did we get to that state in the first place? When we seek help from a medical doctor, they are not extensively trained in the field of psychological development, and they don't have the time to listen to our most profound thoughts that lead to our emotional issues or the state of our heart. Expecting them to be able to fix depression when the cause isn't a physical issue, will continue to lead us down a road of defeat when it comes to depression.

The physical symptoms of depression are often said to be caused by a chemical imbalance in the brain and are treated with a drug based on this symptom. We can't merely take medication and expect our depression to be healed. The cause must be dealt with if we want our mental health to improve or change permanently. Medication might help to relieve some of the symptoms we are experiencing but we need to realize medication alone is not going to cure our depression. As a society, we have become lazy and accustomed to fast food convenience expecting all of our answers to be given to us in a prescription. Life can be hard, and sometimes we have to make changes that we might not necessarily want to make. However, if we are going to improve our mental health and live a life free of depression, we need to take action to make choices that are healthy for us as individuals.

If your job, living situation, environment or relationships are causing you to experience toxic emotions continually, you may have to decide to change the way you are reacting to those circumstances or leave that situation altogether. Our mental health is just as important as our physical health, and we need to be wise in determining what we allow to effect our emotions.

If we take this approach to our mental health on a daily basis, this will protect us from experiencing long-term mental health issues.

When we begin to understand ourselves, we will naturally be drawn to the people who are like us, and we can learn to grow into the person we were created to be. We will begin to love ourselves, even when the people around us are not showing love towards us.

If you're unhappy, maybe you don't know who you are, and you are trying to fit into an environment that doesn't understand you? When we try to put a puzzle together, and we put a piece in the wrong place, it doesn't fit, right? We need the right parts in the right areas for the puzzle to be completed.

Chapter 2: How to Activate and Access the Power of the Vagus Nerve

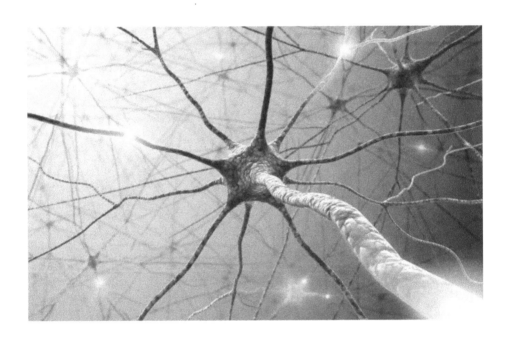

Human Energy Layers

In Divine Love spiritual healing, it does not matter how an illness is contracted or where it is located in the physical body. Removing the harmful energy that causes illness is important, however. That energy can exist in multiple layers and at various locations in the body. The harmful energy is intertwined with the energies of the soul, the mind, and the physical body.

Harmful energy attracts additional harmful energy. When the harmful energy builds up to a high enough level, it is difficult to remove through healing modalities that do not use Divine Love.

Everyone's body has hundreds of energy layers, both inside and outside the body. The first layer in a healthy person is located outside the body about 4 inches from the skin surface. Ordinarily, the body heals energetically from the outside to the inside of a person's core being. Each energy layer is capable of interacting with thoughts and actions.

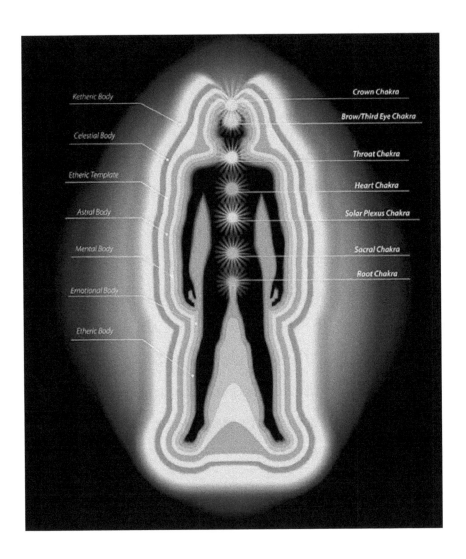

The layers expand and contract as a function of breathing and wellness. When a person breathes in, he compresses his layers toward his core; when he breathes out, his layers expand to their normal position. A person experiencing mental or

30

emotional trauma may project energy layers several feet from the body. Or, energy layers may collapse on one side of the body, frequently causing severe pain.

When energy layers are allowed to expand in an uncontrolled fashion, we begin to absorb emotional energy from other people that can adversely impact our own energy layers. Over time, when someone has severe emotional problems, the layers can become very dense "clumps" of emotional energy that can also prevent proper functioning.

The healing approach used for these two distinct problem sources is very important. We found that about half of all illness cases manifest from stored emotional energy. If these emotions are not released, over time they will literally "plug" your energy layers.

When energy layers become plugged, cells lose their ability to communicate with each other. The cells may die, they may begin to mutate, or they may interrupt body functions. This process eventually produces a variety of symptoms that can become life-threatening diseases.

People may or may not be aware of their energy blockages. Blockages caused by post-traumatic stress may be complex; other illnesses are more easily recognized when they originate from a purely physical cause. An underlying cause can be introduced at any time in a person's life, even genetically introduced at conception.

Activating the Vagus Nerve

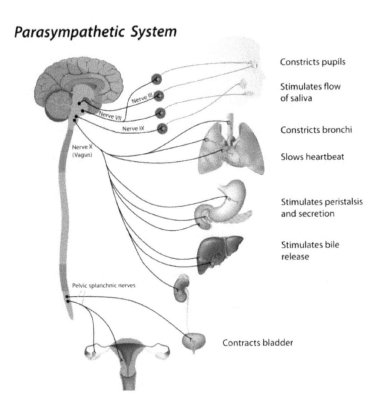

Parasympathetic System

Constricts pupils

Stimulates flow of saliva

Constricts bronchi

Slows heartbeat

Stimulates peristalsis and secretion

Stimulates bile release

Contracts bladder

Divine Love, the universal energy from the Creator, exists everywhere in a neutral state. When you initiate a petition, your spirit activates the energy of Divine Love and then your spirit utilizes Divine Love to effect a change in your body. Your spirit works with Divine Love unless you disconnect from Divine Love before your healing is complete. Should this occur, Divine Love returns to a neutral state and nothing more happens until you reconnect your system to Divine Love. Now you understand the importance of always staying connected.

Harmful energy can exist in some or all of your energy layers. When dealing with a systemic blood disease or sepsis, it is likely that all layers have been contaminated by the harmful energy causing the illness.

For those of you exhibiting major inflammation in your body, you should note that there is a spiritual basis for this. Your spirit and mind interact and cause energetic and physical friction, resulting in inflammation (and sometimes swelling) that does not go away. People with weight control problems will see improvements when they use petitions correctly to eliminate the inflammation in their bodies.

Occasionally, people report that their symptoms return after a few days. This usually occurs either because they stopped the petitions before healing was complete or they disconnected from Divine Love.

Staying Connected to Divine Love

Let us first understand what is meant by accelerated healing. There are three fairly obvious factors to consider:

- When you have multiple illnesses, it should be obvious that it will take longer for you to heal than if you had just one straightforward problem. If you are very ill, it may take your body significant time to process the energy of Divine Love in your body.

- A person comfortable with the spiritual healing process and who has a single symptom frequently experiences instantaneous healing. Others may take anywhere from hours to days to achieve the same level of healing, so please don't compare your progress to others. You are a unique individual and your Spirit knows exactly what needs to be done.

- If you are distracted or become unloving towards yourself or others, you may unknowingly disconnect yourself from Divine Love, and then all healing ceases. Healing does not resume until you re-initiate that Divine Love connection.

By always staying connected to Divine Love, you will transition your entire system into a spiritual mode where you will be living a life of Divine Love. What does it mean to live life this way? Very simply, even when chaos erupts around you, you will be able to function without being driven by your emotions. And, you will be able to function with clarity while others become upset and lose their objectivity.

Also, each time you audibly state your intent to reconnect to Divine Love, you enable Divine Love to bypass any resistance to change that may come from your subconscious mind. This is vitally important to facilitate healing.

Remember that if you perceive that a physical symptom has left or is diminished, but it suddenly returns, it is quite likely that you have disconnected from Divine Love.

Feeling Divine Love Energy

If you are experiencing energy healing for the first time, you may not know the many ways Divine Love energy feels in your body. You might feel heat, a tingle, a vibration, a cooling effect, or even see swirling energy around your body; it is all normal.

Since everyone has angelic support, some people find it more assuring to ask their angels to assist them in processing Divine Love. Years ago, we always invited the Angels to participate. Now, with the energy of Divine Love so high, Angelic participation is optional. Choose to work whichever way brings you the most comfort.

The simple act of accepting Divine Love fills your body with the right amount of Divine Love energy to heal your system. There is always enough Divine Love for the most complex healing, so you no longer need group support. You are self-healing in conjunction with the Creator's Divine Love.

Chapter 3: Vagus Nerve and Anxiety Disorder

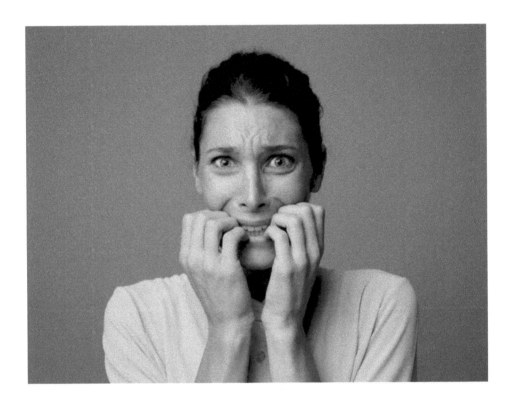

Anxiety Disorder has been misunderstood. First, it is produced from the body. Preconditions are first set by the body and then the mind can enforce it. Of course, a trained mind can make it easier to cope with an anxiety disorder as it is in an out of balance state. The body cannot find the equilibrium between the relaxation and stress modes.

The anxiety caused from the mind will continue by itself for a month because the body and mind will get used to the new psychological fears and a healthy body will find a way to go into relaxation mode. I would emphasize a healthy or well-functioning body, because only when the body is healthy will it find the way. It is designed to go into relaxation mode. No help is needed. And body-induced anxiety will keep it longer, maybe years. The easiest way to treat it is to treat the body.

Many say that anxiety disorder-caused symptoms are the effect of the anxiety itself. Phrased differently, mind-triggered anxiety is the cause and the body symptoms are the effect. But it is not so with body-triggered anxiety disorder. It is both the anxiety and body symptoms that are caused by the body not being able to find equilibrium. Anxiety and body symptoms are both effects of something else, which is the cause.

For instance, a simple example is a small hiatal hernia (in the stomach) which irritates the vagus nerve. Thus, body is the cause and the mind follows. The other way is also true that psychological stresses will bring physiological symptoms. But it will not go for long. It will be stabilized soon.

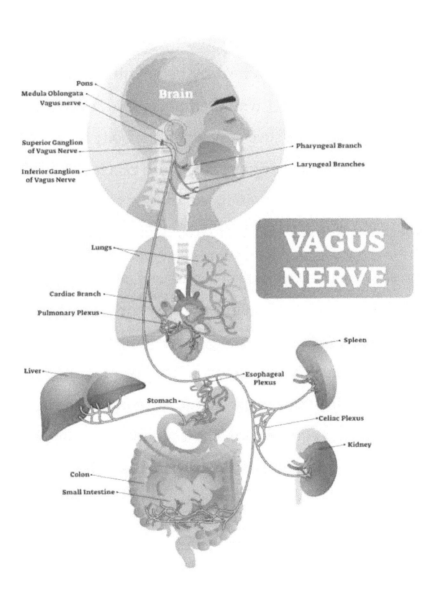

The nervous system that maintains the balance between anxiety (fight or flight) and relaxation can be considered as a loop. Most of the organs are connected to this loop and are guided to operate into two modes: 1) fight or flight and 2) relaxation.

This loop is comprised of the vagus nerve and the nerves coming from the spinal cord. The vagus nerve itself is comprised of two branches: the dorsal branch and the ventral one (polyvagal theory).

Mind-driven anxiety is a broken balance in the mind due to psychological causes. And body-induced anxiety is a broken balance in the periphery (spinal and vagus nerves). The nerves can be disturbed in their path. They can be pinched. The vagus nerve travels a long path which begins from the medulla, located in the brainstem, to all the organs. It is the longest cranial nerve. Thus, it is logical that some muscular-skeletal pressure can affect the vagus nerve along its path. Based on experiences of osteopaths and physiotherapists, the most vulnerable places where the mechanical pressure can happen to the vagus nerve are two: 1) atlas-axis joint and 2) hiatus in the diaphragm (hiatal hernia).

Atlas is the upper cervical vertebrae, also known as C1. The misalignment of atlas can put pressure on the part of the vagus nerve that is located there. When the suboccipital muscles are stiff or tense, the atlas-axis joint can't function properly. A well-qualified osteopath or chiropractor may address the misalignment of atlas.

And as mentioned, vagus nerve irritation also can come from a hiatal hernia. In this case, the stomach puts pressure on the vagus while it goes through hiatus. A well-qualified osteopath or chiropractor may address the hiatal hernia.

The symptoms of a compressed or pinched vagus nerve are too many and manifest differently in different persons. The most common of symptoms are: anxiety, nausea, heartburn, tachycardia, vertigo, headache, a feeling of a lump in the throat, cold hands and cold feet, diarrhea, constipation, sweating and many others.

The vagus nerve can be compressed or irritated at the diaphragm area. The diaphragm can be tensed or become tender. Abnormal breathing, or a slouched position may contribute to the creation of trigger points in the diaphragm. Trigger point therapy or osteopathic diaphragm release may help to release the tension and eliminate the trigger points located in the diaphragm.

First observe if your anxiety depends on your postural changes of body. Notice how your anxiety behaves when you are sitting or standing up and slouched. Try to notice if changing your neck position can decrease the anxiety. Most anxiety disorder cases are due to mechanical causes which may compress or pinch certain nerves. Nerves play an important role in blood supply by dilating the blood capillaries.

It is important to stress that many people have bodily symptoms without anxiety. In such case, the vagus nerve is not involved in these symptoms. Only when the anxiety follows the bodily symptoms the chances are high that the vagus nerve is involved directly in the scenario where the vagus is responsible for all. It would be normal to have mind-induced anxiety directly following some new symptoms but not continuously all the year. The person will get used to the symptoms after some time. Thus, if the anxiety repeats continuously following the bodily symptoms then it is body-induced anxiety where the vagus nerve is involved.

The first step to help the body recover is to do some gentle exercises. It is better to begin for the first 3 months with the *Ping Shuai gong* three two-times a day then to combine with or switch to the *Zhan Zhuang* exercise. *Zhan Zhuang* is the big secret.

Biking is also a very helpful exercise for anxiety but should be associated with an internal qigong exercise. External exercises are good to burn stress but after doing them, they leave us exhausted, while internal exercise, on the contrary, leave us refreshed and energized.

We wanted to say that if you know that the cause of the symptoms is the neck, then you have to treat the neck. If the problem is located in the abdomen, then you have to focus on the abdominal massage, to treat the abdominal trigger points. But when you don't know the cause then it is better to exercise the *Zhan Zhuang*. Moreover, it is typical with the anxiety disorder then usually the symptoms are located elsewhere different from the cause. The pain is here in a part of body but the cause of the pain is far away. The symptoms of anxiety disorder are tricky by misleading the sufferer and the doctor.

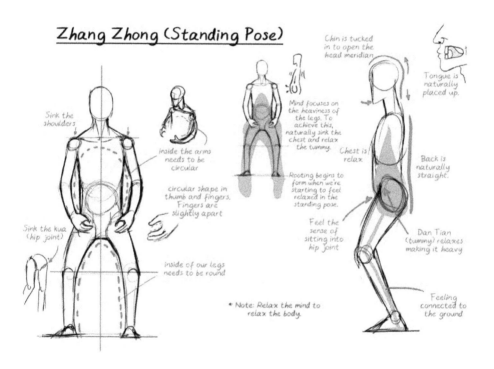

The *Zhan Zhuang* will enable the body to build new neural pathways by giving the body new ways of communication of information through electromagnetic medium. Start the exercise for as few as 15 seconds at the beginning as you are not used to it. And then gradually increase the time to at least 15 minutes. 15 minutes is the minimum for seeing noticeable improvements. 20 minutes is better. The healing process starts at 15 minutes and the max time to practice is 40 minutes. Keep in mind not to exert the body too much. It is important that the upper body remains relaxed.

Whenever you experience new symptoms, it means that your body is experimenting new neural pathways for achieving equilibrium. So, the setbacks and the new symptoms are indications of healing. The healing process is not a linear process. It goes back and forth. Further, the healing effect is accumulative which means in the beginning the results seem to be non-existent, but after some time the healing appears instantly.

Chapter 4: Body and Mind Connection

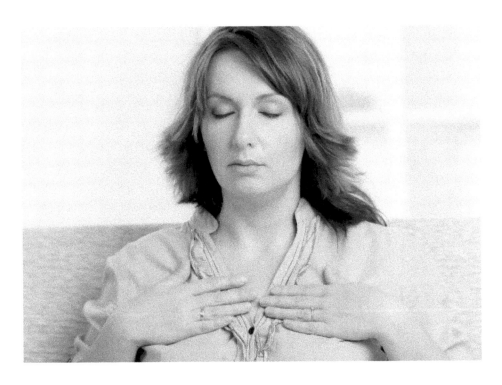

The profound idea that consciousness and matter are interwoven stems from an enlightened mind, as our individual consciousness is interwoven with our physical body. Our individual consciousness is the result of a coherent whole of the body (including the brain). Our individual consciousness is a byproduct of the quantum-interconnected whole of the body, which in turn is quantum-interconnected with the entire universe.

The tendons are comprised of twisted collections of collagen bundles, each of which is composed of collagen fibers. In other words, tendons are part of the connective tissue system or the liquid crystalline matrix. The crystalline structure of the collagen molecules that make up our connective tissue has the property of semi-conduction, as explained in the previous chapter. As connective tissue, our tendons are semiconductors and are able to conduct information, in addition to energy or electricity.

Another aspect of connective tissue (which includes muscles and tendons) is its piezoelectric properties. A piezoelectric substance can convert mechanical energy into electricity. The tendons' piezoelectric properties are nearly the same as those of a quartz crystal. By stretching the tendons in your body, you can thus convert mechanical energy into a DC field or direct current, which is also known as *Chi*.

Many of the tendons in our body are components of the so-called meridians or energy channels. Stretching properly opens the meridians and allows the chi to flow freely.

As for how opening the meridians can be understood, our insights are as follows: As part of the connective tissue, meridians have a liquid crystalline structure. The higher the crystalline structure of the meridians, the better they convey energy and information.

Stretching all of the meridians can improve overall health. The main meridians are connected respectively to different organs of the body. Stretching a particular meridian improves the physical health of organs associated with that meridian. However, stretching all of the meridians makes the body more efficient, as doing so enhances the coordination of all of the organs. More open meridians increase intercommunication within the body and the efficiency of a coherent whole body.

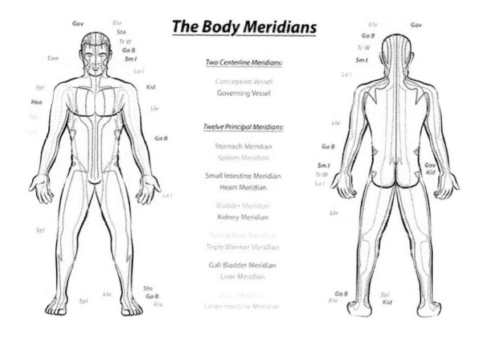

The Body Meridians

Two Centerline Meridians:

Conception Vessel
Governing Vessel

Twelve Principal Meridians:

Stomach Meridian
Spleen Meridian

Small Intestine Meridian
Heart Meridian

Bladder Meridian
Kidney Meridian

Pericardium Meridian
Triple Warmer Meridian

Gall Bladder Meridian
Liver Meridian

Lung Meridian
Large Intestine Meridian

Qigong practices include methods for leading or guiding the *Chi* with the mind. In principle, this practice is very simple. Whenever the mind or awareness focuses on the body, the *Chi* follows. In other words, sensing a particular part of the body causes the *Chi* to travel to that part of the body. Practically speaking, however, such practices should be conducted with the assistance of a master, as inexperienced individuals can disturb the natural flow of *Chi*.

The way of Tao is not a discipline, but rather refers to a spontaneity that emerges by going with the natural flow of things and the wholeness. The philosophy of Lao Tzu cannot be practiced. Whenever you attempt to practice it, you miss it. In fact, the philosophy of Tao is not actually a philosophy, but rather a natural way of living. We will continue to refer to it as a philosophy anyway. The philosophy of Tao differs from Taoism as a religion. The religious form of Taoism came into being approximately one hundred years after Buddhism was first imported to China.

However, the *Zhan Zuang* exercises cannot be regarded as a true discipline, as they aim to open paths for *Chi* to flow naturally by being in tune with the body as a whole. We do not aim to guide *Chi* to a particular area of the body by stretching, but rather to create conditions that enable the natural flow of chi and that foster the body's wholeness. To add to others' hypotheses, we suggest that chi may serve as the direct current, or DC field, inherent in the liquid crystalline medium of connective tissues and the myelin sheath of nerves that enable instantaneous intercommunication throughout the body.

Not only do higher implicate orders organize the lower ones in physical reality, the lower ones also influence higher orders.

Thus, it doesn't matter whether or not you believe in Zhan Zhuang exercises; doing them will improve your consciousness.

Chapter 5: Understanding Chronic Pain and inflammation

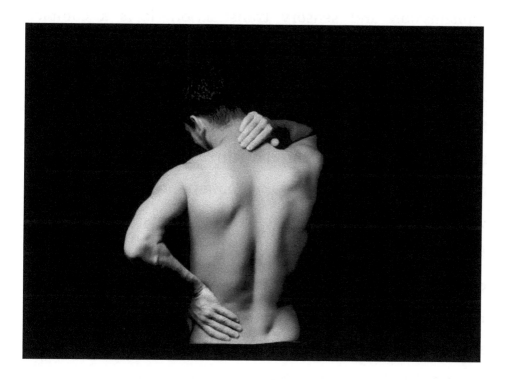

What is Pain?

In actual context, pain is not always associated with physiological processes. Medical attention can identify and treat physical pain, but there's also another kind of pain which is really hard if not impossible to treat through medical means - emotional pain.

So, what is pain? Pain, to put it simply, is far more than neural transmission and sensory transduction, it is a complex mixture of emotion, sensation, culture, experience and spirit.

There are many variations of chronic pain, and it can be hard to distinguish one from the other without understanding its root and consequences. Chronic pain can be upsetting, and lead to a more serious problem when not attended to at once. You will learn that pressures do not only bring about chronic pain from the external environment, but are also an aftermath of certain processes and chemical reactions within the body. Before anyone can appreciate how aromatherapy works to alleviate pain, he or she must first be familiar with how pain is produced and the way the body reacts to it.

When you cut yourself, blood oozes out and there's a sharp pain that follows. If you have a migraine, you feel a chronic throbbing pain in your head. If you are burnt, pain is intensely unbearable. These are different scenarios where a person undergoes a painful experience. Pain in varying degrees of intensity and frequency is identified.

There is a rationale behind the body's ability to sense pain without mistaking it for another sensation. Each part of the body has a function to perform, and those that deal with pain can be influenced to either enable the body to increase its tolerance to pain, or get rid of pain itself. Aromatherapy targets these senses to offer relief from pain and restore overall wellbeing. Aromatherapy also works against the other symptoms associated with chronic pain, and against other conditions linked to the same sensory nerves that produced chronic pain.

Pain can be classified into specific categories based on different factors. It may also be termed acute or chronic depending on the intensity of the pain.

Acute pain is usually milder and is caused as a result of a sudden onset of pain which will go away in a short period like within a few days. It may be caused by damage or injury to the tissues of the bone, muscles or organs. This pain is usually referred to as the warning pain that tells the body and the brain that something is not right and needs attention. This pain is most commonly accompanied by stress and anxiety. These pains can easily be treated using anti-inflammatory pills or muscle relaxants and pain-killers.

Chronic pain lasts for a longer period and is resistant to pain-killers and other medications. It is usually associated with severe anxiety, stress, and other psychological changes as a result of the physical injury. It generally lasts longer and, in some cases, also relapses frequently after an apparent period of relief. Some of the most common types of chronic pains are from arthritis, fibromyalgia, and osteoporosis among others.

What is inflammation?

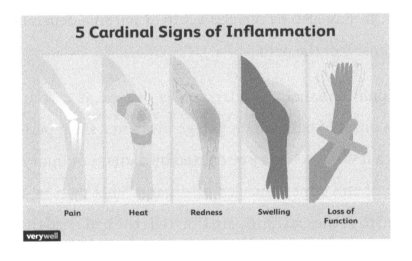

58

Inflammation does not just happen, it is induced by various causes. After all, it is your body's way of reacting to things it finds harmful. Stress puts your body on high alert and enables you to go into a fight-or-flight response whenever you are in danger. However, when your body releases adrenaline, it puts stress in your organs. For example, your heart rate increases and you start sweating or even trembling.

When stress is temporary, stress hormones will definitely come in handy to relieve the situation. But if you are constantly stressed out, the emotional and physical toil on your body becomes too much as your body strives to mitigate all the symptoms of stress.

Psychological stress affects your body's ability to effectively regulate the inflammatory response. It is associated with diseases such as heart disease, depression and various infectious diseases. It weakens your immune system. If you are stressed, you will become susceptible to things such as the common cold. Thus, you should find healthy ways to de-stress. This will lessen inflammation.

Pathogens are another cause of inflammation. Pathogens are basically any agent that causes disease and they exist all around us. Pathogens such as fungus, parasites, bacteria, viruses and mold trigger inflammation when they invade the human body.

Your body induces a natural immune response by attracting white blood cells to the area. These cells work to engulf the pathogens and render them inactive. However, if pathogens such as bacteria and viruses multiply faster than your body can deal with them, then the infection turns into disease and this enhances the inflammatory response as your body struggles to repair the damage. As such, it would be wise to take care of your body, observe hygiene and keep up with your health checks.

Toxins cause havoc in the body. They are poisonous. They work to disrupt hormones, damage organs and tissues, create autoimmunity, cause inflammation and suppress the immune system. Chemical toxicity has been linked to various inflammatory states such as lupus, hepatitis, scleroderma and nephritis.

In order to heal your body, you need to minimize your exposure to toxins. Toxins can be found in the air you breathe, the water you drink and the food you eat. They can also be found in medication, cleaning products, beauty products, mercury fillings, PVC containers and cigarette smoke.

It is important to note that toxins build up in your body over time. Thus, the more toxic products you are exposed to, the greater the buildup. Things such as air pollutants, pesticides, household chemicals, herbicides, food additives and perfumes can all increase the likelihood of inflammation.

Remember, inflammation is basically your body's response to anything it deems harmful. Toxins do not belong in your body and hence, your body reacts to them by inducing inflammation. Stay away from such things.

How Does the Body React to Pain?

The way your body reacts to pain is entirely different when compared to normal stimuli like touch, ordinary pressure and temperature. When the stimulus is non-painful, normal somatic receptors are the first to act. If it is a painful stimulation, nociceptors are the first to fire up.

This pain hinders the body from functioning normally as the mind consistently focuses on the injury or the sensation associated with the injury. Pain exists at different levels:

- **Core response:** This is the first signal that the body transmits to the brain that it is injured and needs help to recover or function properly. This is done to draw attention to a problem.

- **Awareness**: This is the second level of pain and it is the physiological response sent by the brain to the body. As soon as the cognitive portion of the brain receives the signal of the body - it acknowledges it, focuses on it and amplifies it.

- **Emotion**: The third level of pain is emotional concern over the physical pain which can be seen in an inability to accomplish day to day activities normally. This level can also amplify your pain to a greater extent.

- **Social**: This is the last level of pain and it greatly affects your social behavior. This entails a change of mood, attitude and behavior when in pain. This level can also amplify the perceived pain by multiple times.

Understanding your pain is the key to relieving it

Like an alarm clock that wakes us up or a smoke alarm that gets us out of the house, pain is a gift and a friend. Physical and emotional pains are signals to do something that, if ignored, become more intense. Your pain wants recognition and attention. It always arrives with an important message. To find patterns in your pain, document when it happens—what foods, activities, medications, or emotions might be associated with its occurrences. Once patterns are discovered, you are able to experiment with changes that may short circuit the pain reaction even before it starts. Prevention is the best cure of all!

When dealing with physical and emotional pain and fear, this strategy borders on miraculous. The instructions are simple;

the effect profound. It is taught in many mindfulness practices such as yoga, Tai Chi, Qigong, etc.

- First, go to a spot where you won't be interrupted. Do this process alone the first few times, at least, as focus is required.

- Put your awareness, your attention, on the pain.

- Then, allow yourself to feel the pain without doing anything to stop it, to resent it, to fear it, or to change it. Just notice it. Allow it to be. Allow yourself to be with it.

The effect of simply placing attention on a pain or fear can, sometimes, eliminate it instantly. I have experienced that with migraines, tight muscles, and dental pain. An entrenched discomfort often undergoes a change in location, intensity, type of sensation pressure, itching, and heat/cold or other sensations may replace sharp pain. Sometimes, it takes a few minutes for the emotional self to process the physical alteration, to believe it has happened. Even pain that is part of an ongoing situation, a wound, a disease process, or a dysfunctional pattern can become more like "distant thunder" than like an ever-present screaming smoke alarm. The resulting relief allows better sleep and less stress which promotes better healing and coping with conditions. When you get good at this practice, you'll be able to do it anywhere.

Chapter 6: How Pain, Stress and Anxiety Affect Your Life

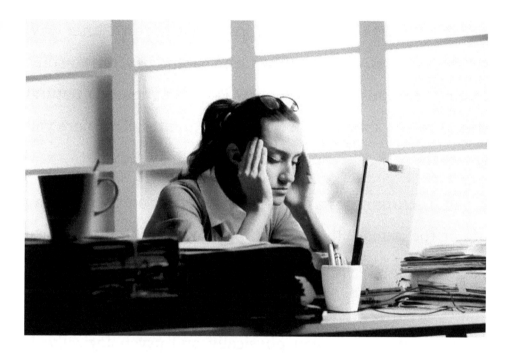

How pain affects your life

At least 100 million Americans, or one in three, live with chronic pain. It's a debilitating condition that affects your ability to work, exercise, focus, relax, do basic household tasks, get a good night's sleep, and fully enjoy life.

Pain can affect your life in numerous ways. If you are a professional and have to go to work, if you experience pain, your work is affected. You will not be able to concentrate on finishing your tasks if something is wrong with you. If you are sick, you have to be absent for treatment or rest. Either way, your work is still affected. If you are a parent, how can you take care of your kids if you are hurt? Pain, is of course a natural stimulus that should not be taken for granted. The more you ignore the pain, the worse your situation may become.

If pain is chronic, it has a detrimental effect on the everyday life of the person. It affects the patient's ability to perform natural functions and responsibilities, and leads to a limitation in physical activities.

Chronic pain affects you physically and psychologically. It limits what you can do. It interferes with your ability to work, play with your children or grandchildren; it also diminishes your ability to take care of your own self. When these happen, pain causes you to feel useless and incompetent, making you succumb to a depression. People with chronic pain often experience irritability, anger, depression, and difficulty in concentrating. It becomes as debilitating as the pain itself.

Chronic pain pressures the person while he is trying to hide the pain and forces himself to cover the handicap by a sense of forged well-being to be functional.

Chronic pain is unpredictable. It is sometimes mild and other times, it is unbearable. When a person is in pain, his perception about things are obscured and his responses are slow. This is the stage where a person's personality does not reflect accurately to the outside.

Pain causes sleeplessness and mood swings. Chronic pain leads to painful depressions and helplessness which, in turn leads to suicidal tendencies, anxiety and panic disorders.

If you're in chronic pain, do you notice the effects that it has on your mood and ability to live a normal life? If you have a loved one who suffers from chronic pain, have you noticed changes in them since their pain began?

Chronic pain has become a large-scale public health issue that dramatically worsens quality of life for many people and creates a sizable and growing financial drain on our health care system. The core of the issue is that the medical community does not know how to address the underlying cause of most chronic musculoskeletal pain. Why are drugs and surgery, which are effective roughly 50% of the time, their go-to treatments? The answer that "these are the best solutions we have" is simply not good enough anymore.

People who are in painful situations are always misunderstood. Oftentimes, their real perception and intentions are not reflected on the outside. Their ways of coping with pain is essentially vital to how people view them. Their view of life is also affected. Those who suffer from serious illnesses perceive life as something they have to live to the fullest as their time short. Some also become hopeless and afraid of the things to come.

The first stop for many pain sufferers is the drugstore, just as the first step for most doctors is to write a prescription for medication. The number of emergency room visits due to overdose of prescription painkillers increased by 34% in just one year between 2016 and 2017. Larger doses of painkillers, often sought by those whose addiction has increased their tolerance for the drug, can cause breathing to slow so much that respiration stops altogether, resulting in a fatal overdose. There are now more overdose deaths involving prescription opioids than there are deaths involving cocaine and heroin combined.

When the structure of the body is damaged beyond the point that rest and improved movement can allow it to repair itself, surgery is typically the best course of treatment. But when function is the issue—as is the case with most people who have chronic musculoskeletal pain—studies consistently indicate that physical rehabilitation is the better choice. It has a higher rate of success, is less expensive, and has far fewer risks than surgery or medication.

To shift out of the surgery-focused trend, some big changes are necessary. Doctors must be educated about the effectiveness of preventive care compared to surgery, and communicate this to their patients. Insurance companies must start covering more types of preventive care. And as a patient, you need to do your part by educating yourself about your condition and getting opinions from multiple doctors. You should also recognize that in many cases there are no magic pills or surgeries that will cure your pain forever. You must put in the work required to take care of yourself on a daily basis so that you can get out of and stay out of pain.

Imaging studies show that regions of the brain involved in making emotional decisions are also involved in chronic pain. To explore this connection, researchers at Northwestern University Medical School and SUNY Upstate Medical University paired chronic back pain patients with healthy control subjects on the Iowa Gambling Task, a card game that measures emotional decision-making abilities. The chronic pain patients performed poorly compared to the control subjects, showing the negative impact chronic pain has on your ability to make decisions.

Another major challenge is that people suffering from chronic pain tend to feel like they have no understanding or control over their pain. Despite all that modern medicine knows about the human body, the medical community still understands relatively little about pain—so much so that 85% of lower back pain sufferers receive no definitive diagnosis.

How Stress and Anxiety Affects Your body and Life

There can be situations when you just cannot act like before you used to because now anxiety its grip on you. It is the feeling of being afraid of the unknown. On a broader sense, anxiety comes in different forms like feeling worried, apprehension, nervousness, or feeling like everything is going out of control. Severe forms of anxiety can be extremely devastating and can have a great impact on your life and health.

Fear and panic are natural human emotions. Everyone has felt anxious for one reason or another. It is the feeling of worry, apprehension or panic in response to certain situations which is usually unsafe or uncomfortable.

Anxiety is a basic human emotion. Generally speaking, it is healthy and manageable to a certain degree. Because everyone experiences anxiety, it can be challenging to recognize and accept anxiety as a problem, however if you just ignore the symptoms of anxiety, you miss the chance to understand your life and yourself better. If you try to understand what your anxiety is telling you, you will have a better chance of overcoming the problem. In effect, you get to enjoy a better quality of life.

Is your anxiety helping you or has it become excessive and detrimental? We'll now try to learn more about anxiety and what you can do to help control the problem.

There are several 'listed' disorders that are all classified as 'anxiety.' Depending on the duration of the anxiety and its severity, it can actually lead to physical symptoms. When it manifests physically, it can cause the person to feel worn out, rundown, fatigued, it can cause pain in muscles and joints, it can lead to an increased risk of getting sick, and it can even increase the risk of heart attack, stroke, and a number of other health emergencies.

There are probably plenty of things that you have gone through in your life that caused you some level of worry. Maybe you had a test in high school that worried you. Even if you studied and felt confident that you knew the material, you might have worried about that test.

Maybe it kept you from getting a good night's sleep right before that test. Would that be considered anxiety?

It all depends. Since it interfered with your ability to sleep, some people could have been diagnosed as having mild anxiety. But most likely once the test was over you were able to get back to your normal routine and didn't worry about it anymore, and that wouldn't be classified as anxiety. More like stress.

We all experience stress throughout our life. It's quite natural and normal, but when you begin to worry excessively about certain things, especially things that you cannot control, then it becomes a problem.

As you deal with stress on a regular basis, whether it's because of financial pressures, schooling, relationship problems, worries about your job or finding work, or anything else, it can develop into anxiety over time.

What usually happens is that the worry starts to consume your thoughts. You begin thinking about the challenges you're facing on a regular basis. You could be thinking about the rent that's late while driving home from work knowing you can't possibly pay it right now.

You could be worried about the company you work for downsizing. You might be concerned about your adult child's well-being because he's out partying every night, doesn't seem to be taking any responsibility for his life, is getting himself into debt, and nothing you say or do – aside from paying those bills for him. -is making a difference.

When you try to fall asleep at night, when the TV is off and everything is quiet, and you can't shut the worry and stress off. You keep turning those fears over and over in your mind.

At some point in the middle of the night you might finally drift off to sleep but the alarm blares just two or three hours later. Now you're tired and have the deal with another day like that.

Multiply that night after night and the anxiety will continue to build even more because now you're trying to focus at work, impress the boss, or getting impatient with people around you.

You might snap at somebody then feel bad about it right away, and that's going to make things worse in your mind. Eventually you may feel tightness in your chest, shortness of breath at times, and have a difficult time getting anything done.

Over time you might withdraw from some of the activities you used to enjoy because you're spending all of your time worrying about everything, even though you're not actually able to do anything about them.

In time, you're living a completely different life with little to enjoy. That can lead to depression and a general state of worry about many other things, even those things that weren't a major concern for you in the past.

Chapter 7: Mind and Physical Illness

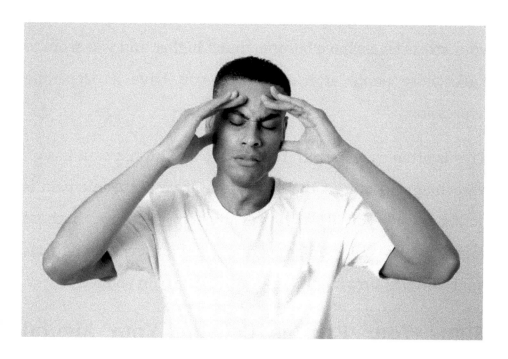

It is not unusual to have both chronic pain and mental issues. These two things are often related, and you need to become aware of how one can affect the other.

It is natural to feel some mental anguish when in physical pain. This is because the mind and body are interconnected and influence each other greatly. An injury sustained on any part of the body, even on an area as small as a toe, can leave you feeling anxious, worried or distressed and the mind then cannot function optimally.

If you deal with chronic pain, you may eventually notice that your stress levels have become much higher and you seem to have more panic attacks, and/or you have a deepening depression.

This is often caused from the effect that chronic pain has on your mental state. At the same time, if your chronic pain is acting up and you already have anxiety or depression, those mental issues could be aggravating your pain, even though it is your mind/brain's mental response to the pain you feel.

Signs Your Pain is Causing Your Mental Issues

You may be wondering 'how will I know', if there is a link between my actual chronic pain and mental issues. The short answer is that you may never know if there is a direct link, if you have chronic pain and a mental issue simultaneously.

However, if one did not start until the other did, there is a good chance they are connected. The good news is that if you resolve one, it might help resolve the other.

But, if you get a handle on your chronic pain, and your anxiety or depression still continues, you should seek out help for your mental issues as well.

What You Can Do About It

The best thing to do is see a professional to get both issues treated.

Physical and mental issues should be treated equally, both conditions are just as important to your overall well-being.

Don't put off getting help for mental health conditions because you don't think they are that serious, or that you can simply do it yourself. Maybe you can, but be honest, after a reasonable amount of time, if the issues persist, get some professional help!

Anxiety sufferers also remember their pain as being worse than it actually was. In studies of people undergoing dental procedures, those who had the highest levels of anxiety before the procedures not only reported higher levels of pain than control subjects, but were also the most likely to overestimate their pain three months later. Sadly, their unrealistic memories of the pain only serve to increase negative anticipation, making their next dental procedure even more painful.

Depression and Pain

People suffering from depression are often unable to take pleasure in activities they once enjoyed, and stress is part of the reason. Stress and the resulting release of glucocorticoids affect pleasure pathways in the brain, raising the threshold needed to perceive pleasure. A stressed lab rat temporarily becomes depressed, requiring stronger than normal stimulation of its pleasure pathways to elicit a sense of pleasure. Based on this research, you might guess that people taking synthetic glucocorticoids as medical treatment would experience an increased risk of depression, and you'd be right.

The effects of negative emotions on pain perception can be induced even in healthy control subjects with no chronic pain and no depressive symptoms. One study asked three groups of volunteers to read statements describing positive, neutral, or negative moods. The volunteers were then asked to try to experience their assigned mood.

As with pain and anxiety, the pain-depression relationship goes both ways; depression worsens pain and chronic pain can cause depression. The two conditions often maintain and exacerbate each other. Suffering from pain that never goes away is enough to make even the most cheerful person begin to have a negative outlook on life. Combine being in pain with the stress of missing work, the inability to do everyday activities, and feeling of being socially isolated, and a mood disorder seems almost inevitable.

To top it off, people in chronic pain rarely get a full, restful night of sleep. Research shows that sleep deprivation reduces your ability to control your emotions and makes you overreact to normally neutral situations. A healthy person feels grumpy when they don't sleep well for a night or two, so just imagine what months or years of inadequate sleep can do to your emotional state.

Chapter 8: The Natural Healing Power of Your Body with Self-help Exercises and Techniques

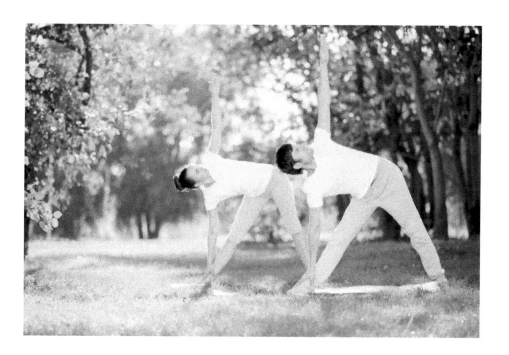

Exercise

Exercise is a necessary part of healing from chronic pain. You don't have to become an active bodybuilder or an athlete, but some degree of body movement is highly desirable to prevent chronic pain. Body movements release the "stuck" energy in our body and ensure a smooth flow of energy to prevent any pain.

Exercising is a great way to reduce your anxiety. Whether you wake up earlier in the morning before you have to go to work and go for a run, or if you can go when you get home from and jog around the block.

Also, if you do exercise more this will help with your self-esteem. Exercising will make you healthier and you will feel better about yourself. If you are worried about your health and it is making your anxiety worse, get out there and do some exercises. You don't even have to leave your house; you could just find an exercise DVD and start doing some exercise from your own living room. To really help lower anxiety, it is a good idea that each time you exercise to be sure it is for 30 minutes or more. Studies have shown that it takes about thirty minutes for your anxiety to lower when exercising.

If you don't want to exercise alone, grab a friend to do this activity with you. This will make you happy and you can have someone to talk to about the things you are anxious about. It's great to have someone who you can let all of your feelings be expressed to who can help you. Healthy exercise has some surprising implications for those with anxiety disorders and other psychological conditions including depression. The mechanisms by which exercise and mental health are related are not fully understood, but many medical experts around the world now acknowledge that exercise has a major impact on a wide range of psychological conditions. It is even now believed that exercise can be as effective at combating depression as many commonly prescribed drugs.

Short bursts of activity a few times a day are the type of exercise that experts recommend. A brisk walk lasting only ten minutes is believed to be enough to raise your emotional state for a couple of hours. For those with anxiety disorders, it can be hard to get out and about on occasion. For some, with severe conditions, it can seem impossible. Exercise, however, will really help to improve your emotional state and take your mind off anxiety. Use the following tips to increase your chances of successfully incorporating exercise into your life.

Moderate level intensity exercise is recommended as perfect for improving your physical health and also your mental health. This includes; walking briskly, cycling, jogging or swimming. Walking and jogging should not need any investment and if you're uncomfortable alone, partner up with a friend or relative. Ideally buddy up with someone who is addressing the same issues or has a good understanding of them, for extra support.

When we exercise, the brain releases endorphins, or "feel good" chemicals that are responsible for the "high" that many people feel during and after exercise. Another benefit of exercise for those with depression is that it lends purpose and structure to each day. Outdoor exercise has been shown to be especially effective for lifting mood.

Regular exercise can help maintain a healthy weight, which can be a problem in depressed people. Exercise promotes overall wellbeing, including heart health and a toned, more muscular body. The weight-bearing aspects of exercise prevent the body from losing bone mass and decrease the risk of osteoporosis, a particular benefit for women.

People who suffer from anxiety may not be interested in exercise. When someone is overwhelmed by the stress of everyday life, working out seems less than appealing. However, research shows that exercise plays an important role in reducing anxiety symptoms.

While exercise has been clinically proven to reduce anxiety and improve mood, it can also treat a number of other health problems. Health issues can be a major anxiety trigger, and easing the symptoms of those ailments can reduce anxiety symptoms further.

In addition, exercising can help people relax. When a person exercises, their body releases hormones that produce a calming effect. Exercise also increases body temperature, which can be very relaxing. Working up a sweat is tiring, but it's a great way to calm down.

Speed Walking

Speed walking, more often referred to as power walking or race walking, is a technique of walking at a rapid pace. Walking is a great alternative to running and is oftentimes much easier and more accessible to a greater variety of people. Walking provides all of the aerobic benefits of running while steering clear of many of the injuries associated with high-impact techniques of running. The activity of walking at an increased rate then walking "normally" can help participants lose weight, tone their muscles, and also increase their mood.

Not only is speed walking valuable for the muscles and joints, but it also reinforces overall health.

Stretching

Stretching is something everyone should do on a regular basis, and those with chronic back pain will benefit most from stretching the soft the muscles, ligaments, and tendons in and around the spine.

It is a fact that when motion is limited the back becomes stiff, which can result in more pain. Those who suffer from chronic back pain need to stretch regularly and perform appropriate stretching movements to benefit from the sustained and long-term relief from the increased motion.

One top recommendation for dealing with chronic pain is by getting regular exercise. Exercise will help with different types of pain - from helping with arthritis by getting your body moving, to boosting your mood, when you have pain from Crohn's disease or fibromyalgia.

Yoga for Chronic Pain

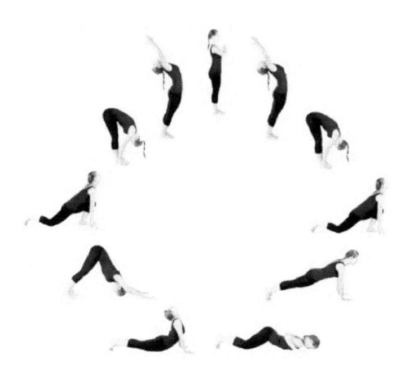

Yoga can be defined as a practice based on harmonizing the mind, body, and soul. By practicing Yoga every day, you will not only explore your true self or your inner self, but also develop the feeling that you are one with nature and environment. Yoga aids the overall well-being of the body and focuses mainly on developing relationship with the natural world around us.

Pain is not just influenced by physical injury or illness, it is also greatly affected by our thoughts, anxiety, trauma, stress and emotions. Stress and pain are closely interrelated - you may experience pain when stressed and stress can also increase the intensity of the pain. When there is increased stress, your breathing becomes heavier, erratic and ragged. Your mood is also altered along with some tension and tightening of the muscles. These symptoms of chronic pain can even increase the toxins in the body and decrease oxygen levels.

Yoga addresses these problems effectively, as it involves the techniques of deep breathing and meditation, which helps in the absorption of much-needed oxygen and also in the relaxation of mind and body. These breathing techniques ensure that the muscles of the lungs, diaphragm, back, and abdomen are fully utilized. When the muscles are loose and relaxed, they can help in releasing the built-up tension in the body and facilitate proper flow of energy throughout. Stress and anxiety levels will also be reduced gradually.

Yoga, or simple stretching, are simple practices that should be applied to everyday life to reduce the tension of stress and keep the muscles in proper working order. There are specific stretches that can focus on problem areas such as the neck or lower back. These stretches can be assigned from a personal trainer, massage therapist, or physiotherapist. Yoga can be enjoyed at home or in a studio with several other participants. There are many forms of yoga ranging from hatha yoga to hot yoga. The focus in yoga is on breath control, meditation, stretching, and balance. Not all forms of yoga are spiritual with chants and mantras, if you don't feel comfortable with that form of practice.

Exercise in general is good for chronic pain, but specific exercises, especially certain yoga positions, help to decrease some types of pain, like shoulder or neck pain.

Additionally, the relaxation techniques you will learn, can teach you how to manage the different types of chronic pain more effectively.

If you are considering trying yoga techniques for your chronic pain, you need to consider the style of yoga you will do.

While all forms of yoga can be beneficial for your body, mind and spirit, certain exercises are actually directed towards people who are struggling with chronic pain.

There are multiple yoga poses or asanas and different stance can be used. Individuals with chronic pain should begin with a slow-paced, gentle yoga pose. Benefits of yoga include improved ability to handle stress, feeling more relaxed throughout the day and improvements in sleep quality. Studies have proven that yoga is helpful to prevent fibromyalgia, among other chronic pain conditions.

Massage Therapy

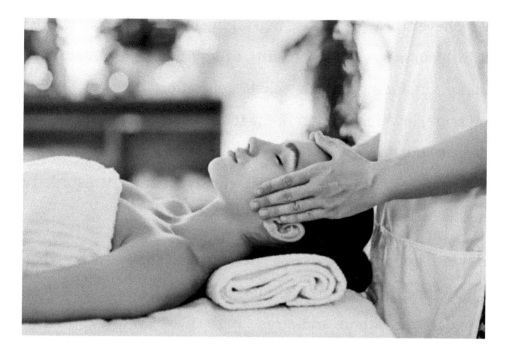

Massage therapy has become overwhelmingly popular, and rightfully so; in addition to feeling good, it has a number of health benefits. Massage therapy is wonderful for any type of pain, be it chronic, acute or simply from fatigue, work, and tension. There are various massage therapies available to meet all types of needs, including Shiatsu, Swedish, hot oil and deep tissue.

Massage has also been used as a natural anxiety remedy for ages; it may be as simple as rubbing your neck gently but whichever the case you are massaging it is an effective way to calm your nerves. The benefits of any massage therapy are many, including stress relief, relaxation, lowered blood pressure, lowered tension in the muscles, and it also improves deeper breathing. As the book unfolds, I will discuss therapeutic massage as a natural remedy for anxiety disorders, in this case it will be a deep and precise tool.

A skilled and trained massage therapist will know exactly what to do once the pain problem is explained. Massage also does wonders for fatigue and stress, both of which are known to increase pain and go hand in hand with arthritis and other chronic pain conditions. It can also help to calm anxiety, which often afflicts those who suffer from chronic pain.

If you can afford it, get a massage regularly - weekly or even twice per week. Physical therapists and chiropractors also offer therapeutic massage, so it may be covered under medical insurance.

There are also electronic massagers on the market that are great options. These include mobile units, which are spot massage products that target the neck or specific areas. There are also strap onto chair units that offer *shiatsu* for the entire back, many come with a heat option.

The most significant health benefit of massage is that it provides the sensation of touch, which is critical in both early childhood development and overall adult health. Levels of somatotropin, or human growth hormone, correlate directly with the amount of physical contact you receive.

Massage also cues relaxation in your nervous system. One of the biggest benefits of massage is that it feels great, especially if you're in pain. Nerves that carry information about the sensation of touch to the brain are more heavily myelinated than the nerves that carry information about pain, so touch information travels faster than pain information. This is why you instinctively rub the skin around a painful area; the touch sensation temporarily drowns out the pain sensation, and you're given a brief moment of relief.

Massage also feels good because it temporarily reduces muscle tension. Pressing on tight muscles lengthens them in the same way that gentle prolonged static stretching does, and after an hour or so of this manual lengthening you may stand up feeling like your muscles are made of jelly. If your massage therapist applies a great deal of pressure, your stretch reflex may be activated immediately, making you feel tight and sore soon after a massage. A good rule of thumb is that if you feel pain during a massage, you're probably going to feel some soreness afterward as well. While it can be difficult or awkward in the moment, it's better to ask your massage therapist to press more gently than to suffer the consequences. It is absolutely not necessary to apply a painful amount of pressure to reap the benefits of a massage. Moreover, if you're in pain, a deep massage can increase and prolong your pain by making your muscles tighter.

Lastly, massage temporarily softens connective tissues, which increases flexibility and range of motion. Tendons, ligaments, fascia (which surrounds, supports, and separates structures of the body), and scar tissue (which forms to heal an injury) are all made of collagen fibers arranged in varying patterns and densities. As muscles become habitually tighter and movement decreases, connective tissues also respond by tightening. Movement and heat can make these collagen structures more flexible and fluid.

For people with chronic pain, the most beneficial aspect of massage may be that it lowers stress, thereby reducing the sensation of pain and reactivity of the nervous system. However, a massage by itself is not enough to change deeply learned habitual movements or your resting level of muscle tension. The sensory awareness that can be gained through massage is valuable, but if it isn't followed by actual motor education in the form of voluntary movement, little lasting progress will be made. You must actively retrain your nervous system, and you can't do that with massage alone.

Brain Balance

First, you have to make sure your brain is balanced. Without a balanced nervous system, your efforts to eliminate chronic pain will be wasted. Many things can cause brain imbalances. Most common are head injuries and exposure to electromagnetic radiation from personal wireless devices. Things that increase brain imbalance risk factors include:

- Using Bluetooth devices and cell phones, walkie talkies, using desktop and laptop computers and iPads.

- Eating processed foods that have MSG.

- Consuming drinks containing artificial sweeteners, and drinking fluoridated water.

- Leading a stressful life.

- Not getting enough quality sleep.

Brain Balancing Using Affirmations

Studies show that when the thymus gland is balanced, both hemispheres of the brain also remain balanced and serve to lower chronic pain. The nice thing about affirmations is that they don't cost you anything; you just have to repeat the affirmations regularly throughout the day to keep your brain in balance. You need to "feel" the words to get full benefits. The following is a list of daily affirmations:

- I have faith, gratitude, trust, love and courage.

- I'm modest, I'm humble and tolerant.

- I'm clean and good, I deserve to be loved.

- I'm content and tranquil.

- I have forgiveness in my heart.

- My life energy is high, life is full of love.

Brain Balancing Music

Brain balancing music encourages a balanced nervous system and balances both hemispheres of the brain. Brain balancing music uses three coordinated methods: "primordial sounds", "brainwave entrainment", and "multi-layered music" to bring the mind-body into a deeply relaxed and balanced state. You have to listen to the music on a daily basis to maintain your brain balance which is crucial for health and healing of chronic pain.

Avoid GMO foods

GMO or genetically modified organisms have been introduced to our diets over the past decade. As of this writing, the GMO foods are not labeled in the U. S. So, the average American's is unconsciously consuming GMO rich canola oil, sugar. beets, corn, soy and cottonseed oil. GMO foods can cause all sorts of gastrointestinal problems, allergies, weight gain, and immune problems. Avoiding GMO foods can reduce or even eliminate many health problems, including chronic pain.

Emotional Freedom Techniques

This amazing technique deals swiftly with all sorts of emotional pain and has an infinite number of applications. EFT has been around for quite a while and is now used in many hospitals and psych units throughout the world by professional psychologists and psychiatrists who are continuing to get very positive results with severe emotional pain and trauma.

There is no doubt that strong emotions can be very painful things and it is now recognized that emotion follows thought. This is why psychiatrists spend years talking about trauma and trying to uncover triggers and thoughts that cause bad feelings, depression, phobias and the like.

EFT is a great way to deal with all fear though you will have to be thorough. Really take a look at all the different aspects of that fear and treat each one with a very specific opening statement.

Emotional Freedom Technique (EFT) or tapping requires that you tap specific acupressure points on the torso, hands and on the head in order to clear energy blocks caused by negative emotions and feelings.

What you do is tap lightly on each of them. You get used to doing this very quickly, and when you have been using EFT for a while you can just do a few taps here and there, maybe on your collarbone or under your eye, for rapid relief.

Generally tapping involves two stages. In the first stage you are tapping to express the negative emotions. This stage of tapping will last as long as you have an emotional charge, continual tapping will bring that charge down to a minimal level.

The second stage includes reframing the condition positively where you choose a positive emotion or thought to replace the negative ones. The cool thing is you can't tap incorrectly; your intention is enough to make it work correctly. Even without tapping the right acupressure points, you will still release the negative energy from your body.

Basic EFT instructions

Choose a negative emotion or feeling you wish to clear based on a situation that is troubling you. For example, you might be angry at your neighbor Tom for letting his dog poop in your backyard.

First, feel where in your body the negative emotions are contained and tap there. This may be one location or many. When you feel your emotional charge has dropped significantly and want to move on to the positive rounds, then tap all the acupressure points again and review your state of feelings. For example, as you tap, you might say, "I choose to be open", "I choose forgiveness", "I choose to let go and move on",etc.

Cultivating a Positive Attitude

The easiest way I know to create a positive attitude is to count your blessings. I know, I know, that may sound like old hat, something you've tried a hundred times, you think there's nothing to be thankful for, but look closely and start really small.

First of all, concentrate on small things then you will find them extending out, past the current moment. Remember, start small, if you have beautiful strong nails, list those, if you like the way your old slippers keep your feet snuggly warm, list those. Become aware of the tiniest pleasures throughout the day and mentally add them to your list.

Now do that three times a day. It only takes moments. You can write them down if you wish. First thing in the morning, lunchtime and before bed. Make it a rule and do it for at least a week.

So, the goal is to create an attitude of gratefulness, for what you DO have, and in this way, you open the floodgates for a whole lot more of the same. Whatever your beliefs on the subject it is an inescapable fact that like attracts like, whether that is misery or joy, so you may as well choose joy!

Visualization and Setting Goals

Visualization and setting goals are important. You should have one big goal – to fully heal and return to normal, or an even better life – and some small milestones you will set for yourself. Visualizing a life where you are pain-less and is free to do whatever you want can help in cementing your determination to heal. This will also keep you up when the emotionally-taxing treatment brings you a bit down. By setting a final goal at the end of smaller goals, the big one feels easier. This is achieved by slowly traversing through the smaller goals one by one. Set a daily or weekly goal and visualize what you will be able to think and do by the end of that time period. Always give yourself some time to feel the celebration of your accomplishment for every milestone. Not only will it give you a needed break in your climb towards betterment, you will also feel more encouraged to go on and reach the final goal.

Guided imagery, or creative visualization as it is commonly called, is another alternative therapy that can be used in pain management. This method involves focusing the imagination on certain positive events or behaviors that you would like to occur in the future. The principle behind this practice is that the mind and the body are connected and they influence each other. The emotional trauma associated with some physical injuries and events can be replaced by these self-suggestions, positive images, and creative imaginary techniques.

Many researchers have stated that visualization is one of the most effective and powerful tools of change. It can have great positive impact on the patient if guided correctly. Visualization can be done independently or under another's guidance. But most researchers opine that it is more effective when somebody else guides you through the process as you respond more quickly to the guidance of an external voice.

There are numerous ways to start the process of visualization. If you are practicing it independently, there are many CD's available online and in retail outlets that can guide you through the process.

Utilizing visualization for pain management is a powerful technique. By doing this, the brain starts to respond to the inputs given in the form of two-dimensional images. Then the brain sends out the signal for the body to relax. Therefore, by imagining the situation where you don't feel any pain, the body relaxes as the brain starts responding to those stimuli. This technique is very effective in treating different types of health issues both physical and emotional.

Visualization should ideally be performed in a quiet area where you will not be disturbed or distracted. It is best to keep the lighting dim or even maintain total darkness. Each of the sessions may last from 20 minutes to an hour and you may start feeling slight positive changes from the very first session.

Music Therapy

Music therapy offers numerous health benefits, but it is frequently used for physical and mental pain management. It helps to relieve stress and anxiety, which is often exasperated by pain, as well as giving you a mood boost when you are experiencing chronic pain.

It should create a gentle and relaxing response in the person listening to the music, which if done right, can help them reduce their pain or at least help them handle it better.

With just a little research, you can experiment with music therapy on your own, or seek out a licensed musical therapist who has gone through a training program.

Your music therapy program might include listening to music or getting you involved in making music, writing songs, or just singing along to songs.

There are several reasons to give it a try.

- You may not need to use as much pain medication, which can cause other body issues, can become addictive, and eventually stop working.

- If you find it is helping, add it to your anti-pain arsenal, as it is a good, ongoing therapy that can help with long-term pain management.

- The fact that it can reduce stress and help your body relax, is often why it often works for chronic pain management.

- This will help improve your overall quality of life - naturally.

- Find a professional to learn more about music therapy if you would like to explore this natural method for helping with your chronic pain.

Comfort yourself

Comfort and give advice to yourself as if you're helping your best friend, or a close family member. You are your greatest friend and your closest family after all; just as you are your worst enemy. It works both ways, you know. Of course, such an activity that requires clarity of thought and focus of your mind requires that you, yourself have identified what exactly is wrong. So, dig in and help that pain-filled, trembling you inside that is experiencing a darkened interior of your heart.

Letting Go

It is very painful to blame yourself for something that you have no control over. Guilt and self-judgment is one of the leading causes for chronic pain symptoms and are usually either self-imposed or are drilled into someone throughout a significant period of time. It could also be an experience long gone in the past that no one can do anything about anymore. In such cases, letting go would be the best option. One cannot totally forget memories, especially those that are heavy enough to cause impacts that affect you physically in the present. But they can be accepted, acknowledged and regarded as valuable stepping stones for the current you to reach where you are now. Don't endanger the future for something that happened in the past. Let them be your inspiration, your motivation to keep moving forward and up, instead of taking them with you like shackles that remind you of the pain. Don't live in the past, gradually move on into the present and be hopeful for your future.

Biofeedback

Biofeedback is a special technique that helps people to improve their health conditions by training them to control certain involuntary processes of the body. Using the biofeedback mechanism, the individual learns to change his physiological activity in order to improve health conditions and performance levels.

You may think biofeedback is not a self-help technique to eliminate chronic pain, but it is really an effective method. Biofeedback is helpful for everything from gastric distress, high blood pressure, migraine headaches, anxiety, sleep disorders and muscle pains. Biofeedback is generally done under supervision of a health professional, but with a little training you can do it yourself. Basically, biofeedback involves listening to a relaxation tape and having a small electrode taped to one of your fingers.

Biofeedback sessions can take 15 to 30 minutes and during that time you will be using guided imagery and relaxation breathing. While you are practicing relaxing methods, you can see your heart rate or skin temperature in the monitor.

The therapy involves attaching electrodes to the skin, which displays the results to a connected monitor and this is the information that is used to help control your involuntary functions. There is no exact evidence on how the biofeedback technique works, but many experiments conducted by researchers have reported that it gives relief from stress and helps the body to relax, which is vital for maintaining good health.

Relaxation Training

Relaxation training involves employing some innovative methods of stress and pain management. The techniques are geared at helping you keep up with your day to day activities with ease. Relaxation is not just enjoying a good movie or watching a game, relaxation happens when both mind and body are calm, de-stressed and in-sync with each other. The best part about relaxation training is that it is free of cost, takes relatively little time and it can be practiced anywhere. Whether you are travelling or sitting in the office, you can spare a few minutes to unwind. The goal of this relaxation therapy, like any other alternative therapy, is to avoid the use of traditional medicine and treat the problem as naturally as possible.

Meditation and Mindfulness

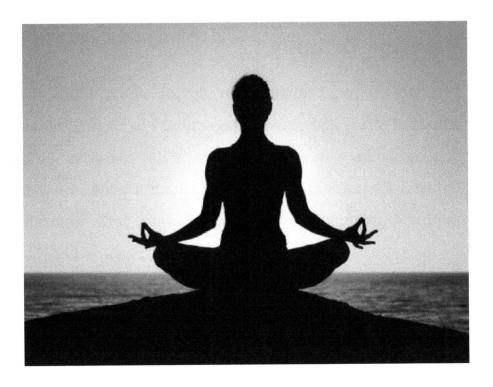

It is human nature to worry, but when those worries consume and inhibit you and your daily life, then you know it's time to take control of your mind. Meditation is a highly effective tool to re-center your head and control your thought patterns. When you are trapped in your head with anxious thoughts, your brain is conditioned to think negatively. Your automatic reaction is to think of every worst-case scenario. This is a vicious cycle, and one that may seem impossible to break. Don't be discouraged, you have the power to demolish your inhibitions and take back your mind.

Meditation allows you ample time with yourself away from listening to what everyone is telling you about your condition. Every time you are anxious, take a deep breath and maintain a steady relationship with your breathing and take notice of your surroundings, the natural sounds around you and your body's response to the stimuli being introduced to your senses.

Meditation is a practice wherein a person induces an alternate level consciousness or trains his mind to practice stillness. There are a variety of techniques for promoting relaxation, establishing stillness, and building internal energy. When you meditate, you relax your mind and body. Meditation should be done in a quiet and peaceful place in order to attain peace of mind. You can do meditation alone or in a group.

Meditation can offer profound rest to your physiological self by activating a parasympathetic response in the nervous system, also known as the relaxation response. Essentially, rest is a natural way of getting rid of anxiety and stress. Your body is designed to eliminate stress when you sleep.

Today, there are a lot of stressors around. You can get stressed out from your daily activities, the people around you, and the situations that you are in. If you want to have a healthier mind and body, meditation may be the relief you have been looking for.

Simply put, meditation is the practice of awareness. It is awareness of your thoughts, your body, and who you are. Meditation involves ridding your mind of the abundant chaos in the outside world, and focusing on the condition of your own spirit. It is easy to get caught up in what is happening externally, and meditation teaches you who you are aside from your racing thoughts. There are different ways to practice meditation, all of which focus on different types of mindfulness. All of them are beneficial in overcoming anxiety.

Meditation is broadly known to help with pain management and relief. Unlike the methods already mentioned, meditation brings relaxation, clarity, and healing to the whole self without any particular focus on specific components or issues.

Meditation makes minds, intuitions, and bodies operate more efficiently. Combining this with whatever level or kind of yoga you can tolerate will enhance the benefits of each.

Meditation can be described as a state of deep peace that occurs as a result of a calm and stress-free mind. What you will discover, however, is that the peace and serenity that you find during your meditation sessions, carries over into other areas of your life when you are not actively involved in meditation.

It has been proven that stress and anxiety are at the root of many health issues. When you integrate meditation into your life, it will lower your stress and anxiety levels, boost your morale and reduce the pain symptoms associated with psychosomatic conditions.

The practice of meditation requires some amount of discipline and a willingness to persevere. Only the most rigorous of meditators can successfully train their mind to concentrate for long hours at a time. However, you do not have to aspire to meditate like a Zen master to reap the benefits of meditation. You can start with shorter sessions of perhaps ten to fifteen minutes and slowly increase the length of each session. You can practice anywhere and at almost any time. There are some techniques that are discussed below that may integrate well into your regular activities and allow you to practice often.

Many relaxation techniques and meditation exercises can be combined with an ongoing TMS treatment. By meditating, the patient can better explore their psyche and emotions as well as relaxing the body to let go of the involuntary tensions. These usually cause the pain and fatigue that are characteristic to psychosomatic disorders. Chronic pain sufferers tend to think "this will go on forever", "I'll never get better" or "I'm no good for anything anymore." By meditating on the positives and encouraging oneself, such hurdles are crossed and stresses are released, readying the mind and body for the healing to set in.

Commonly known as meditation, it's now mentioned as mindfulness meditation or integrative medicine because it's relieves a wide range of chronic diseases, stress and pain. Studies have shown that mindfulness is an effective technique to increase brain activity and physical changes to increase antibody production. Therefore, it is a must-use method to include in your daily schedule. Mindfulness lowers the production of stress hormone cortisol and decreases the need for pain medications for chronic pain.

Aromatherapy

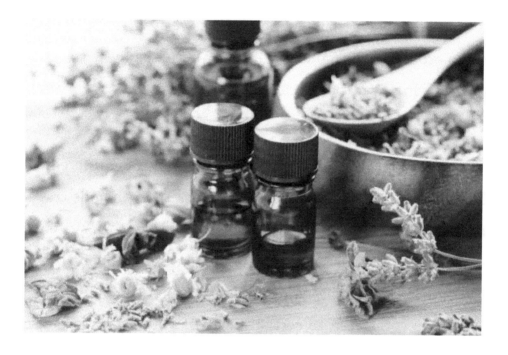

Aromatherapy is a type of alternative therapy that makes use of aromatic plant products such as oils and extracts to treat different health issues. Aromatherapy can be performed using scented oils, fragrant candles, potpourri, or any product that is fragrant and evokes a relaxed, calm feeling.

Essential oils work as natural pain relievers. They have certain properties that facilitate natural healing processes within the body.

Essential oils are derived from organic materials, and are processed in ways that can maintain its very core. In this case, these aromatic substances will not interact badly with other medications; or rather, it can function without aid from other drugs.

When essential oils enter your body, they have incredible healing effects. The fragrance molecules from the oils travel through your olfactory system (one of the sensory systems, responsible for your sense of smell) and make it to your brain to combat those feelings of anxiety and stress. Your limbic system is connected to certain parts of your brain that also affect blood pressure, hormone balance and stress levels. Essential oils can be used topically or inhaled using aromatherapy to soothe anxiety. To add to their qualifications as outstanding healers, your body can absorb and spread their healing powers through your body within five minutes of exposure.

Essential oils are a powerful and versatile way to free your body from anxiety. The aromas and the properties of these oils are essential in your self-care recipe.

Using only aromatherapy as a solution for anxiety will probably not yield quick results, but when used in combination with other therapies, it can be helpful. Here are a few ways you can incorporate aromatherapy for anxiety and stress:

- Essential oil massages.

- Wearing an aromatherapy scent during the day.

- Get a diffuser and have it on during the day. Some diffusers have a light and a timer that will help if you wish to use it to fall asleep.

- If you're in a rush, or as an emergency measure for a panic attack, you can also sniff essential oils straight from the bottle or sprinkle a few drops on a tissue.

Essential oils are a healthy and natural way to calm your body, mentally and physically. The molecules in the aromas of the oils are capable of affecting your brain, and controlling feelings of stress and anxiety. They also have the ability to change heart rate, blood pressure and the function of your immune system.

When essential oils enter your body, they have incredible healing effects. The fragrance molecules from the oils travel through your olfactory system and make it to your brain to combat those feelings of anxiety and stress. Your limbic system is connected to certain parts of your brain that also affect blood pressure, hormone balance and stress levels. Essential oils can be used topically or inhaled using aromatherapy to soothe anxiety. To add to their qualifications as outstanding healers, your body can absorb and spread their healing powers through your body within five minutes of exposure.

Lavender Essential Oil- This is one of the most effective oils in treating anxiety. This oil can improve concentration, calm anger and irritability and also promotes relaxation which combats insomnia.

Cedarwood Essential Oil—An essential oil that promotes the release of serotonin, which is a neurotransmitter in your body that regulates mood. Also, this oil helps regulate appetite. This is beneficial because in some cases, feelings of anxiety can cause loss of appetite. Cedarwood oil also helps if you have trouble falling or staying asleep.

Eucalyptus Essential Oil— The strong aroma of this oil eliminates stress and gives you an energy boost. It is the perfect pick-me-up to get rid of those feelings of sadness.

Rose Essential Oil—Rose oil also boosts feelings of peace and well-being.

Essential oils are a powerful and versatile way to free your body from anxiety. The aromas and the properties of these oils are essential in your self-care recipe. In the next chapter, you will learn how meditation can rid your body and mind of anxiety. You will also learn how you can incorporate the use of essential oils in your meditation practice for an extra soothing experience!

Supernatural Healer

You have the power to set in motion the forces of supernatural healing for your sickness, disease, situation or circumstance whatever they may be. At this point if you have not read the teaching on the "Spirit Realm", it would be wise to do so. Much of what you will learn here assumes that you are familiar with the spirit realm. You will be missing a key step in your quest for divine or supernatural love of God and his intervention in your affairs without an understanding of the spirit realm.

You see, there is a zone where supernatural healing occurs. It is here that the supernatural healer can be reached and it is accessed through the spirit realm in the same way that you gained access to this teaching by getting into this book.

There are certain key truths to commit to mind about supernatural healing. The first is that you must know and believe in the author of supernatural healing – a higher power. It must be clear to you that he is Lord of your life and Lord over every condition that you face. You must also tell him that you believe this to be true.

Because you have become his child, God the father will pay attention to your requests and meet them according to what is in your best interest.

Although man is a spirit being, he lives and operates in the physical realm. However, if you wish to appeal to divine intervention in order to gain control over the issues of your life, whatever they may be, it becomes necessary to gain access to the spirit realm.

In other words, effective appeal to the person of the supreme God and the forces of his dominion and authority, (and they are awesome), can only be offered and accepted in the spirit mode. There is no shortcut and there is no other way to do this. Only a spirit can communicate effectively with another spirit.

Using Outside Imagery

Another technique is to take your mind away from your body. There are quite a few different ways to use imagery, always starting with positive imagery. You want to imagine something that brings you joy, no negativity allowed! Imagine you are pain-free and are enjoying a place you would love to be, such as the cabin you go to every summer, maybe you love to ski and want to feel the fresh snow air, or the warmth of a sandy beach in a tropical climate. Another way to use imagery is by using the pain as a symbol, such as a light bulb. Slowly you want to dim the lights, helping to imagine your pain is gradually lessening. But don't stop there. You are also feeling pain-free, doing activities with that special person. Now, when you come back to your current reality, ask yourself, "Why aren't I doing these things? What do I need to do to achieve them?

Self-Reward

Reward is positive reinforcement, every time you overcome your fears you can reward yourself with something that leaves a mark of assurance and emphasizes that inner voice that keeps telling you 'you can do it' every time you are anxious.

Decompress

Anxiety activates the nerves to quickly react to your fears by relaying messages to your brain and back to your body. Decompression keeps the nervous system in check so that it doesn't run wild whenever you get anxious. Take a warm heat cloth and wrap it around your neck and shoulders for ten minutes, close your eyes and relax your muscles, face, upper chest, back muscles and neck.

Anti-Stress Journal

1.   Write about one incident in your recent past that made you feel stressed.

2.   Record your thoughts, emotions, and bodily sensations: Did you feel angry and blame others? Helpless? Resigned to the situation? Did you feel tightness, pain, or tension in your body? If so, where?

3.   Record the steps you took to address the stress: Did you light a cigarette? Have a drink? Go outside? Call a friend? Slam doors?

4.   Next, record daily stressful incidents and your reactions for a week.

5.   At the end of the week, review the journal and identify your patterns of reaction.

6.   Zero in on one or two reactions that you feel are especially harmful to your mental or physical health and that you want to change.

Research confirms that self-hypnosis can relieve stress. Through self-hypnosis using visualization and imagery techniques, you imagine yourself effectively managing the stress systems in your life. Practicing such techniques on a frequent schedule can help you cope with those stressors on a daily basis.

Detoxification

Activated Charcoal

Recent studies have shown that using activated charcoal from coconut shells is one of the best ways to detoxify. Activated charcoal binds to toxins, chemicals, and other carcinogens and safely eliminates them from the body. This is great to have on hand if you have an upset stomach as well. Hospitals use activated charcoal in cases of overdoses and poisonings. If you decide to begin taking activated charcoal, please note that it will absorb and remove any vitamins and mineral supplements you take, so be sure to take it many hours apart from nutrient supplements. Experts recommend taking 500mg on an empty stomach, upon waking and before going to bed. Coconut shell activated charcoal is recommended because it won't pull needed minerals out of the body. Please check with your healthcare provider to make sure this is a beneficial option for you.

Skin Brushing and Saunas

The practice of dry skin brushing is simply using a dry skin brush to open up the pores of the skin and increase circulation. Skin brushing can be done before getting into a bath or shower. All movements should be aimed at the heart. For instance, brushing the arms should start at the hands and move upwards towards the shoulders, in the direction of the heart.

Infrared saunas are another way to eliminate toxins through the skin. You simply sit in a sauna for approximately 20 minutes and the sweating brings the toxins out of the body through the skin.

Gallbladder Flush

Gallstones are eliminated through the bowels after a brief fasting period along with the intake of Epsom salts, grapefruit juice and olive oil.

It is recommended that you do a liver flush at least once a year, or more often for people who are experiencing severe health problems. This flush helps to cleanse the liver and the gallbladder to help your body eliminate toxins more efficiently.

Grounding

"Grounding," also known as "earthing" is a simple, free way to heal your body and connect with the healing energies of the Earth. This term refers to simply putting your bare feet or body on the Earth. Examples of this include walking barefoot (on grass or at the beach) or lying directly on the grass or sand.

Because of our modern practices of walking with shoes, living in multiple story buildings and using frequency-emitting electronics all day long, we have not tapped into much of the healing properties that the Earth provides.

Self-Hypnosis Training

Self-Hypnosis will allow you to dive deeply into relaxation and give positive suggestions directly to your unconscious mind. Please practice self-hypnosis twice a day for 21 days.

1.   Sit in a chair and close your eyes.

2.   Imagine yourself walking down a flight of stairs.

3.   As you descend, it becomes darker and pleasantly warm.

4.   Maybe you smell roses.

5.   Tell yourself that with each downward step you are becoming more relaxed.

6.   Once you feel calm, imagine yourself turning around and mentally climbing back up.

7.   With each step tell yourself that you are becoming more ready to cope with the challenge that awaits you.

8.   Once you get to the top, say to yourself, "I am calm and capable. I am refreshed and ready." Keep your eyes closed until you feel centered.

10.   Open them and feel refreshed.

Think of a suggestion or positive statement you wish to tell yourself (your unconscious mind)

Spiritual Healing

Negative entities are nothing to be frightened about, but it is important to know they exist, and to have the tools to protect yourself from them. They can be picked up in many ways: from traumas, alcohol or drug use, dabbling in the dark arts, sexual encounters, and many other ways.

Because we have free will, we must be very conscientious about drawing boundaries with what kind of energy we allow in our personal space. If you do not specifically let it be known that you do not consent to their presence, they have "implied consent" to stick around your energy field.

If you suspect that some of your anxiety is stemming from a negative attached energy, you may find it helpful to seek out an energy healer in your area who is well-versed in removing attachments. You can also do this yourself if you wish.

Choose love over fear. Fear and Love cannot co-exist at the same time. A lot of folks suffering from anxiety find their minds focused intently on what they fear. By doing this, you are edging out love. By consciously choosing love over fear, you can start to change your mindset. When I first started this practice, I would start to experience a worrisome thought and then I would say aloud "I choose love." It helped quite a bit and became natural the more I practiced it.

Express gratitude

Being grateful for what you have doesn't just make you aware of how blessed you are in life. It also gives you an appreciation for your hard work and the work of others, and leads to a happier and healthier life. Here's how you can adopt a more grateful attitude to bring about a positive mindset:

- **Write down everything that you are grateful for each day.** You still have your journal from section one right? If so, start listing down the things that you are happy for each day. If you're ever down, reflect on these things and find happiness in what you have.

- **Be mindful.** There are so many things to be excited about each day. With a little mindfulness you can cultivate inner happiness as well. All you have to do is start acknowledging everything that you have and everything you receive on a daily basis.

- **Share your appreciation with someone else.** If someone is meaningful in your life, let him or her know that you care. It's easy to overlook the importance of other people in our lives and it's important that we share how we feel in the time that we're given.

- **Say thank you.** Sometimes that's all you need to do.

If you are prone to anxiety, it is common for you to focus on the negative aspects of your life. The positives are overlooked more often than not. A wonderful way to combat this habit is to write down ten things you are grateful for every single day. You can do this first thing in the morning to feel positive starting the second you wake, which will set a good tone for the rest of your day. You can also do this in bed at the end of the day so you can fall asleep with a smile on your face.

To be honest, there are a million and one ways that things can go wrong in every moment. Your situation could be much worse than it actually is. Try to focus on the good things that are happening in your life. Look for things that you can be grateful for. Do you have a roof above your head? Are there people in your life that make you smile? If you focus on the good things that happen in your life, it is very likely that you will feel less anxious about what the future holds.

If you are currently having a pain in your elbow for example, start picturing one of your feet.

Focus on your foot and what it feels like. How many miles has that foot taken you? How many times have you experienced a wonderful time because your feet got you there?

Say, "thank you, feet".

Crystals and Healing

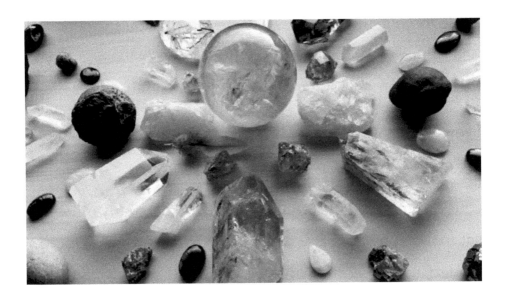

Crystals have a long history of healing on many levels. For centuries, societies have valued crystals for their brilliance as precious and semiprecious gemstones as well as for their unique vibrational energies within each crystal that can help facilitate healing for the body, mind, and spirit. Cultures throughout history, including ancient Roman, Greek, Egyptian, and Asian, used crystals for their healing properties. Sacred texts included information about crystal healing, people buried the dead with significant stones, and warriors and royalty wore crystals on different parts of their body and made use of talismans and amulets for good luck and protection. Ancient acupuncture needles were tipped with crystals to enhance healing. We find ourselves today utilizing similar techniques involving crystals and healing stones.

This technique of healing requires the crystals to be placed on or around our body. The crystals can be placed at specific points on our body or they can be moved over the body in a particular manner that will eliminate the negative energy and bring relief. Even though this method gained popularity in the past few decades, ancient records shows that crystal healing dates back to as old as 6000 years. Egyptians and Sumerians have the oldest records of using crystals to heal the body and bring back balance. Other civilizations who used crystals for healing purposes are the ancient Indians and the Chinese.

We can make use of this resonance in different ways. They speed up our body's healing mechanism by bringing back balance to our energy system. Just like crystals, people are different from one another and that is why the resonance of crystals will guide different types of people to different types of crystals. This resonating with a particular crystal depends upon the state of the body and mind of an individual at that particular moment.

How Do Crystals Heal?

Energy is the essence of everything in the universe, including the human body. In the same way, each crystal vibrates to a specific kind of energy. As you work with crystals, their energy blends with your own, transforming and amplifying the energy within your body. Subsequently, the crystals are also important as they assist in re-energizing and rebalancing your body on the emotional, mental, spiritual, and physical levels.

Normally, each kind of crystal will radiate a particular type of energy that corresponds to and works with the specific energies in certain emotional and physical areas of yourself. Using crystals for healing is as simple as being around them. Other techniques may include holding a crystal in your hand or placing it on a nightstand.

Since these healing crystals are constantly absorbing negative energy in order to provide healing, they can become blocked.

Blockages will then reduce the healing effects of the crystals, hence the importance to cleanse them.

Various crystals have energetic signatures that can be helpful for anxiety. Below are a few of different types, along with their healing properties.

- Covellite (Dark blue) - Known to replace negative emotions with serenity, helpful if you are feeling vulnerable. It releases anything holding you back. Helpful for detoxification.

- Cerussite (Clear, gray or brown) - This stone inspires and facilitates hope and willingness to overcome difficulty and feelings of being overwhelmed, aids in overcoming perfectionistic tendencies. It also increases concentration, helps with ADD and ADHD. It's helpful for anxiety attacks, social anxiety or agoraphobia.

- Gaia Stone (Green) - A reassuring stone that brings harmony, serenity, and calm; banishes nightmares and aids in restful sleep, eases migraines, headaches, stress and gastric upset.

- Lithium Quartz (Lavender/pinkish gray) - Increases calming and peaceful feelings. Reduces the intensity and frequency of panic attacks. It helps people who are currently using antidepressants or other pharmaceuticals.

- Petalite (White, colorless, gray, pinkish or yellow) - Excellent for healing emotional trauma of abuse/ victim patterns. Brings self-acceptance and self-love. Used for ADD, ADHD, excessive worry or stress. Helpful for regulating blood pressure and countering anxiety attacks.

- Rhodochrosite (Usually rose colored) Helps to heal the inner child and emotional traumas. Ideal for nervous system imbalances, as it heals the myelin sheath that protects the nerves. A good aid when withdrawing from caffeine. Has anti-anxiety and anti-stress benefits.

- Blue Calcite (Blue) - Calming, lowers blood pressure.

Since crystals generally have higher vibrations, they are a natural enhancement to meditation practice. When we focus our intentions while gazing at or holding a specific crystal, this increases the power of the energy and intention. You may not feel something right away. Be patient, open-minded, and keep trying.

Crystals are powerful in stimulating a lethargic mind and promotes calmness as well. Crystal can assist in boosting a person's creativity, clarity, and concentration. They help raise human vibration thus bringing focus to your mind. Crystals to use for mind calming and clearing are clear quartz, amethyst, sodalite, bloodstone, and carnelian.

Clear quartz placed above or around the head and crown chakra will provide your body with clearing energy and allow it to get back to its most perfect state of balance. Calming amethyst relaxes your mind and improves your memory, creating focus and concentration. Carnelian can be very activating, letting the mind sharply focus, and dismiss mental fogginess. Sodalite also has a strong effect on the mind. It can eliminate mental confusion and encourage intuitive perception and reasonable thought. This opens the mind to see things in a different manner and to receive useful new information. Bloodstone can be an excellent tonic crystal to relieve an overactive mind. It reduces mental confusion while increasing alertness. It helps in adapting to changing or stressful situations, maintaining mental stability. This helps in clear decision-making. It can be beneficial to keep a bloodstone in your pocket during any type of test or exam, to help focus on a solution rather than a problem.

When energy healing work is done, the energy will align with your highest and greatest good. Sometimes the change you think you need or want is not what best serves you. Get rid of any expectation of the result and allow what serves you to come forth. When we set expectations and stick to them, we limit ourselves and results. What we imagine is usually smaller than what the universe makes available to us. Sometimes what serves our greatest good doesn't appear as we think it should.

Try to remove "should" and "could" from your vocabulary and accept what the energy brings. Sometimes changes are subtle and take a while to occur. Sometimes they are immediate and very obvious. Oftentimes, when major healing occurs, a shift in our reality can throw us completely off balance. Understand the need for change but allow yourself to let go of any expectations of how and what change should happen. Set your intention, do the work, remove judgment and expectation, and be open. The energy will always serve your greater good.

Prayer Healing

We believe that separating the spirit from the body has retarded the healing process of the whole person. In modern times, many medical students emerge from their studies with their sights trained on the laboratory rather than on the examination room. They have been trained as pure scientists rather than as whole-person doctors. As a result, the gulf between doctor and patient has widened. Prayer and positive mental attitudes are often not included in the medical bag. Many physicians consider religion nonessential or even a liability. This scientific exclusiveness may have arisen out of the concept of dualism advocated by the French philosopher René Descartes. The blame for the fragmentation of the human person, however, cannot be placed on scientists alone. Religious leaders have become defensive, and the pulpit sometimes becomes a place for condemning science and its accomplishments.

The art and science of physical healing in modern times has become the responsibility of the medical doctor and other trained professionals in the health-care system. They have been taught to recognize the causes for physical problems and to find ways to assist nature in the recovery process. Through the use of medicine, the doctor has been able to give nature a boost in manufacturing antibodies to combat invading germs. Through the use of surgery, the doctor has been able to remove the tissue or organ that is causing malfunction. Through the use of certain devices and physical therapy, the doctor is able to aid in the restorative process. Each of these methods of healing has benefited millions of people needing help.

Smile heals

As always, laughter is still the best medicine. Induced feeling of happiness or even generally feeling good can do wonders for your condition. Doing fun things, watching funny movies and shows, or even just finding something to laugh at, helps you get over your negative emotions. Have fun with your friends and family. Enjoy hilarity wherever you can find them and practice looking at the brighter side of things.

Laughing is a great relaxation technique and stress reliever. It increases lots of good feelings and serves to discharge tension. One major problem with people prone to anxiety is that they tend to take life so seriously that they appear to be melancholy all the time and they eventually stop creating fun moments in their life. Fun and play are essential for the proper functioning of the brain; it is a technique that stimulates the brain to come up with creative ideas rather than concentrating on unreasonable worries and fears. Within the fun and play you may find various ways to reduce stress that you can apply in situations when you are rendered anxious and helpless. Remember that rigidity limits you to a certain scope of ideas that will directly influence your take on the world.

Have you noticed lately that the times you smiled, you felt good? Sometimes, a smile just appeared while you were thinking about a time, a place, a person, who brought you moments of happiness.

Remember a time, when you saw something, and you just thought it was hilarious. Remember the time you did something and it made everyone in the room laugh. It was not an embarrassment moment it was hilarious moment.

Some people have the ability to make others smile and laugh. You really cannot do one without the other. Have you ever seen anyone laugh without smiling? And when you have a deep smile, you are generally laughing inside.

Just, as there is power in words, you have power in your natural ability to make yourself happy. Although you may never reach the level of a constant state of happiness, it is possible to live totally in a state of happiness and, it should be your desire and goal.

Learn how easy it can be to naturally heal yourself. Sometimes, when your nerves are wrecked from hearing bad news, or because a deadline is approaching, money is short, reserves drying up, phone ringing, dog barking, baby is crying, grandchildren screaming loudly, or "life just happens" and it is the unexpected, you just want peace and quiet. Just laugh to get an instant natural high sensation.

Tap into your reserves and gain control. You have an internal well of happiness if you will only dig down deep enough to find it, even in a stressful situation. Laugh at the moment, it is not as bad as you think. Take a few deep breaths and feel your energy return.

The more we smile and laugh, the more we can temporarily relieve pain from our mind and body. Maybe, if more of us kept the ability to smile that we naturally had in childhood, we would not have to take so many anti-anxiety medications.

Mental Imagery

Mental Imagery is a powerful technique that can help you not just with pain management, but many different areas of your life; such as accomplishing important goals. It helps the speeding up of recovery, pain relief, boosting the immune system, resolving emotional and physical problems, and much more. There is no limit as to what visualization can do for you.

Visualization and mental imagery works because our unconscious mind doesn't recognize what is reality and what is imagination. Therefore, what you imagine IS reality to your unconscious mind. This process involves focusing on the imagination/ visualization whilst being in relaxed state of mind.

Research has shown that stimulating the brain through imagination may have a direct effect on the nervous system and endocrine system, while helping to promote changes in the immune system. Guided Imagery can help stimulate healing by releasing endorphins, which are a natural pain analgesic.

Chakra Healing

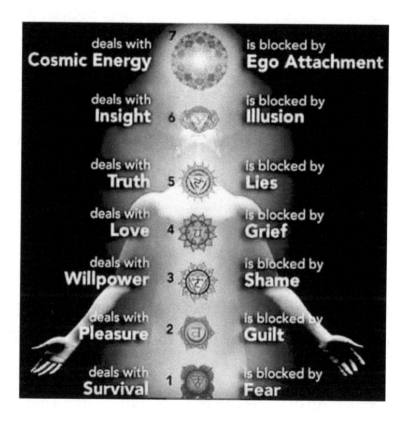

Knowledge of the chakras and how you can strengthen them is vital to your overall physical, mental and spiritual health. Chakras are typically defined as the (sometimes) invisible force fields around you, which emanate positive or negative energies depending on your mood, emotions and health status.

The chakras are crucial to the health of your body. Even if just one of the chakras is poorly aligned, you will notice that all of them can become blocked and not working that well. All of the chakras need to have energy flowing through them properly; so if one of the chakras doesn't allow the energy to flow through, there are going to be some significant problems that arise. You need to learn how to let the energy flow through the chakras to help them to feel better, and this can be done in no time at all.

When the chakras are opened up, you will notice that you feel so much better than ever before. Opened chakras allow you to talk to others, open up your heart to others, feel grounded in the world around you, and even to have a connection to a higher power. All of these can be important to live a happy and healthy life. In many cases, our modern world makes it difficult to keep the chakras working as well as we would like them to. We are too stressed out, we are worried about keeping our jobs, and we may not have much of a chance to open up to other people. It does take some active work to help keep the chakras as open as possible.

There are so many elements of your life that can go wrong when you are dealing with your chakras not working correctly; and if one of the chakras is out of order, and not letting through the energy that you need, all of them can begin to fail pretty quickly. As a result you may not be able to show or share love with other people in your life, or you may not be able to stay grounded in the life that you have.

Another problem that you may have is that a chakra will allow in too much energy compared to what it should. For example, if your throat chakra is open too much, you may blurt out anything that comes into your head, even if it isn't necessary or will cause a lot of pain to someone else when you say things that are not necessary. When the throat chakra is working correctly, you will find that it works well to help you be honest and speak up correctly, so you don't want it to let in too much and say a lot of things that are not necessary and could cause issues with other people.

Herbs

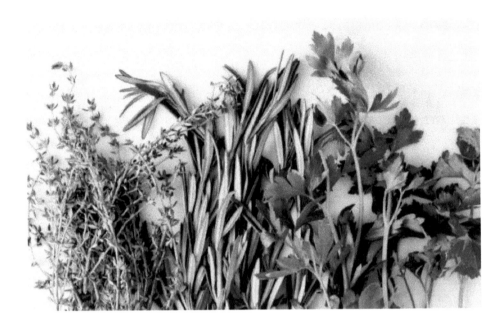

Anxiety cannot really be cured unless the core of the cause that produces it is dealt with. Any herbal approach will alleviate the symptoms but not the disease itself. If those symptoms are not severe to the point that professional care is essential, and you are otherwise quite capable of carrying on with your everyday life, then soothing agents can be used for the symptoms before any medical intervention.

Herbs to cure Pain and Inflammation

These herbs are good if you suffer from pain and inflammation in various body parts or the joints and bones.

Feverfew

This herb has been proven to be effective in preventing and curing migraines. The active ingredient in this herb functions to minimize the serotonin level in your body, while relaxing the blocked blood vessels located in the head. Other migraine-related effects that feverfew herb can treat is reducing pain, vomiting, nausea and high sensitivity to noise or light. It can be particularly effective if you suffer from repeated migraines, to reduce the frequency of the attacks.

For the desired results, take a dosage of about 50-250 milligrams of dried feverfew leaves, equivalent to 2-3 fresh leaves with or without food. You can also make a tincture by dissolving grinded leaves in ethanol. The active ingredients in feverfew include parthenolide and tanetin, which are responsible for the healing properties of feverfew.

Witch Hazel

If suffering from conditions such as hemorrhoids, you can reap the benefits of the anti-inflammatory properties of this herb. Witch hazel has numerous benefits such as relieving itching and the discomfort associated with hemorrhoids, while minimizing the irritation and burning in the rectal areas.

Witch hazel contains active compounds such as flavonoids and tannins, which are volatile oils that act to stop bleeding. The bark of witch hazel is effective in treating internal bleeding through injection to the rectum. The procedure is aimed at reducing the pain and the itching caused by hemorrhoids. For vaginal care, you can cleanse the infected area by wiping, patting, or blotting.

Chinese Skullcap

Chinese skullcap is very effective in treating inflammation caused by arthritis. This is due to the active ingredients such as Baikal skullcap and catechu, which are also known as flavocoxid.

Other conditions that Chinese skullcap can treat are the inflammation of the air passages in the lungs, bronchiolitis, and other lung infections. A combination of Baikal skullcap, honeysuckle and forsythia can be effective for children suffering from bronchiolitis. The condition is usually caused by respiratory syncytial virus infection.

Meadowsweet

Meadowsweet herb has active substances that are included in aspirin, and chewing the roots can help in reducing headaches and other pains. The active ingredients found in this herb include tannins and salicylic acid, substances which your body easily converts to aspirin. Meadowsweet can be particularly important if you suffer from arthritis that contains gastritis, a condition characterized by inflammation of the stomach lining.

The best method of taking this herb is inclusion in teas from herbal extract. The recommended amount of herbal content should be about 4-5 grams of meadowsweet for the herb. You can make herbal tea with 4-6 grams of the dried herb and take the concoction 3 times daily.

Herbs and Supplements for Anxiety

Chamomile

Valium is a common drug that doctors prescribe to help their patients relax. This drug binds to certain brain receptors that help the brain to quiet its processes. This helps people to relax and unwind during the evening, giving them a chance to get to sleep.

Chamomile contains certain compounds that do very much the same thing as valium, but in a much safer, less addictive, and healthier manner. Apigenin is the active ingredient in Chamomile and researchers have found that those with General Anxiety Disorder actually experienced a decrease in their overall anxiety level after taking chamomile supplements for eight weeks.

Valerian

This herb has been known as affective, but should not be consumed for more than three weeks after taking this herb. A side effect from taking valerian could be getting a headache. Valerian is a sedative to the brain and nervous system. You should take valerian before bed, as it is known to make you drowsy. You can find these valerian capsules at your local drug store.

There are some anxiety reducing supplements that won't make you feel sleepy, but Valerian isn't one of them. It doesn't smell all that great, but it's a potent way to help reduce anxiety levels and get you a good night's rest.

When you sleep well, it helps you deal and cope with situations throughout the day more positively and effectively, thus reducing your overall anxiety levels even more.

Passion Flower

You're not going to suddenly fall in love when you begin taking this herbal supplement, but it has been proven to be effective at reducing the level of nervousness a person experiences in certain aspects of their life.

It is considered a sedative and certain research studies have shown that passion flower is just as effective at reducing anxiety levels for people as some prescription medications. So, while you'd be giving your body something natural, you'd also be eliminating the need for those potentially addictive pharmaceuticals that often come with a long laundry list of potential side effects.

Green Tea

L-theanine is more commonly known as 'green tea' and it has been used by people for thousands of years. Buddhist monks relied on green tea and they were able to meditate for hours on end.

L-theanine has the ability to lower heart rate and blood pressure, which can begin to trigger a calmer mode for the individual taking it. There haven't been a high number of research studies on humans taking green tea supplements, but the few that have noted a tendency to reduce overall anxiety levels. However, green tea may not be enough for those with more severe forms of anxiety.

Lavender

This is an intoxicating aromatic flower that can help calm emotional worries. A Greek research study found that patients in a dental office reported being less anxious about their impending visit when there was lavender throughout the room than those who didn't have lavender complementing the room.

Lemon balm

Lemon balm is a great herb to reduce anxiety and is known to even help you sleep. Lemon balm is sold in capsules, tea, oils, and in extracts.

Fish oil capsules

Fish oil is great to help with anxiety. You can find the capsules at any drugstore. They are usually in the vitamin isle. Fish oil does not taste very good, so it is a good idea to get it in a capsule and take it down with water. This will help relieve stress, it is a good idea to take fish oil capsules in the morning before heading out to work. If you already eat a lot of fish, then you do not need to take fish oil capsules. Great oily fish that you can eat to take place of the capsules are salmon, sardines, and even mussels. You want to eat different types of fish which are full of fatty acids to get the proper intake.

Kava Kava

Getting kava capsules will help with anxiety. It is a very powerful herb, so be sure to take this kava capsule every once in a while, do not take it on a daily basis. If you are suffering from anxiety and depression this is a great herb to turn to for help. This herb has been known to drop anxiety and depression tremendously. You can put kava in your hot tea. It tastes really good, but it does make your mouth a bit numb.

Skullcap

Skullcap is very effective for anyone who has high anxiety, muscle tension, and jaw clenching. It is known to help with anxiety, insomnia, high cholesterol, allergies, and skin infections. This herb will be found in a capsule and could be store bought at any drug store or vitamin store. Skullcap is referred to as a mint, so this will also be a great herb to put into your hot tea to help reduce anxiety.

Winter Cherry

Winter cherry is also known as Ashwagandha. It is often taken in a capsule or can be put into tea. It is known to balance your emotions when you have mild anxiety. Winter cherry plays a huge role helping with social anxiety. This is a great herb to consider taking if you have mild anxiety or social anxiety.

Talking therapy

Talking therapy is a blanket term for all psychological therapies that involve a person talking to a therapist. Counseling, cognitive behavioral therapy also known as psychotherapy, family therapy, group therapy and couple's therapy all fall under talk therapy. Depending on the problem one type or more types of therapies may be better suited for the problem than others. In addition, different talk therapies vary with different people, for one person counseling may work best to achieve positive results and for the other psychotherapy is the only way to go. Below is a brief explanation of what each talk therapy entails.

Communication is very important in all treatments, most especially for painful conditions. First, that should be with your doctor or counselor. Making regular updates with your progress can help them assess any need for adjustment and can also encourage you when you are hesitating in stepping onward. Communicating with your friends and family can provide immense amounts of support. Psychosomatic treatments can be very trying for relationships, but the best ones weather through by constant support and understanding. You'll come out of the experience together even closer and tighter than before. Also, communicating with other people suffering the same conditions as you do can be quite a help. It is still quite a different kind of support to give and receive encouragement from people who are experiencing the same things as you do. The feeling of helping others out is also quite a good addition to your self-healing.

Talking therapy is for anyone going through a rough time and can't cope with the negative energy that emanates from it. It is always soothing to have a person who will listen to you, understand you and help you get through. Talk therapy gives room for people to overcome some inhibitions like fear, for some they find it easier to talk to strangers about their problems instead of immediate friends and family members. The sessions in talk therapy usually create a strong connection between the patient, the problem, the therapist and the solution. Patients may not necessarily heal from their anxiety immediately but a therapy session is strong enough to make them think about better ways out of their problem.

Counseling is the best-known talk therapy and the one that is most readily available. You can get counseling from anyone provided they have a good understanding of your situation backed by facts that will help you achieve your goals for the therapy. Parents, guardians, teachers, mentors, religious leaders and friends can counsel you if they are good at it or have in one way or another undergone a similar situation. Professional counseling is normally done by counselors who have actually studied and specialized in this field. Counseling sessions usually take 6 to 12 sessions and each session should be a maximum of 1 hour. Counseling for anxiety disorders requires the person to first acknowledge that the counseling session is for her own good, that they embrace the counselor, understand that no hard feelings should be manifested and she must also be willing to talk her thoughts out to the counselor. Being free with your counselor is the best way to fight anxiety, you are safe to allow yourself to get anxious in his or her presence and anytime you feel you are having an anxious fit you can call them up and talk about the experience.

Cognitive behavioral therapy

The aim of cognitive behavioral therapy in anxiety relief is to help a person think less negatively and instead of them feeling hopeless they start adjusting to situations easily to a point that they even enjoy what they are going through. CBT is a very practical therapy and talk is the central tool used to communicate ideas; you set certain goals with your therapist and in between session you carry out different tasks that exercise your motor skills and how best your cognition relates with them. The minimum therapy sessions that you can attend are 6 and the maximum are 15 with each session lasting an hour. CBT deals with current events occurring in a patient's life instead of focusing on past events, this is another similarity that is shared with counseling. Patients with various mental health problems reacted positively to CBT therapy and the effect improved on other areas of their lives.

Psychotherapy

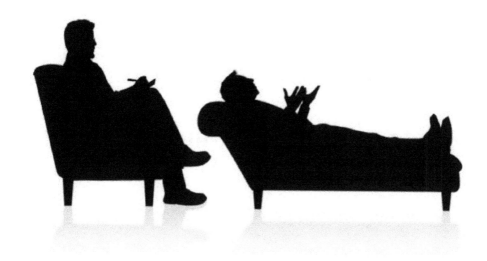

Unlike CBT and counseling, psychotherapy involves an active indulgence in your past events. The therapy seeks to treat current problems by evaluating past events and identifying a connection. Psychotherapists usually listen to their patients relating bits of events from their past and how it affects their present life. This therapy lasts longer than all the other talking therapies and it deals with complex anxiety disorders like post-traumatic stress disorder. It may take the patient longer to go back into memory lane and talk about their experiences as some of them may have been brutal, but with psychotherapy they gradually adjust into their past life experiences and they open up about them. Most psychotherapists normally work from hospitals, clinics and mental institutions and the sessions normally depend on the severity of the problem and the time needed to address it.

Foods to Help You Fight Anxiety, Stress and Depression and Pain

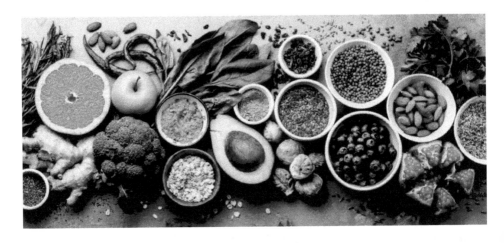

What you eat is very important in how best your body fights the anxiety and its symptoms. First off is to avoid heavily processed foods and unhealthy fats and oils. For breakfast you can have comfort foods like a bowl of oatmeal which is not only good for your heart but is also full of calories to see you through until your next meal. Foods that create some hormonal imbalance in the body must also be avoided at all costs, try complex carbs as an alternative.

What we nourish our bodies with can't be underestimated, as it affects the physical and emotional aspects of ourselves. Many fine books exist on diets for every kind of illness or state of recovery from injury. However, some of these do not go far enough for maximum benefit. In other words, they play to our hope that we can eat and drink what we want and still get healthier.

To be honest, there are many foods that are not going to do you much good, but research has shown that when people are hungry, they are more irritable. When you're more irritable, you're more prone to emotional outbursts and worry.

If you're feeling extremely anxious, it's a good idea to try and eat something to help you relax. Make sure you focus on healthy foods, though, and not something that is bad for your body.

Fruits and vegetables are extremely important to eat on a daily basis, so the next time you're feeling hungry in between meals, snack on some celery, an apple, or some other healthy food and you may very well find yourself feeling more relaxed as a result.

A lot of people don't realize that certain foods can actually lower levels of anxiety. You can start taking control of your levels of nervousness by being more conscious about what you eat. Here are some examples of that:

Foods with Magnesium: Foods that have a lot of magnesium could help with general calmness, such as swiss chard, spinach, nuts, legumes, whole grains, and seeds.

Foods with Zinc: Nutritional sources that have zinc, such as eggs, liver, beef, cashews, and oysters lower anxiety levels.

Probiotic Food Sources: Foods like sauerkraut, pickles, and kefir have been linked to lessened anxiety symptoms.

Some foods are especially good at combating depression and anxiety. Here are several that will help you win the battle.

Eat lots of whole grains

Whole grains are those grains with intact kernels that have not been processed. Look for "whole wheat" and other "whole" ingredients in the ingredients list if you're not sure if it's a whole grain. Whole grain products include whole grain pasta, whole grain bread, brown rice, quinoa, rolled oats, barley, and many others.

Eating whole grains is beneficial because these foods have all of their nutrients still in them. Again, these foods are high in B vitamins, including folate.

Eat plenty of fiber

Fruits, vegetables, legumes, and whole grains are also high in fiber. Eating high-fiber foods can help prevent constipation, a side effect of some antidepressant and anxiety medications. Shoot for 25 to 30 grams of fiber every day from fruits, vegetables, legumes, and nuts.

Whole Foods

When treating anxiety, nothing is as safe and simple as consuming the right foods. A number of foods have natural calming properties, and a number of nutrients can help the body fight back against anxiety. With a diet rich in whole foods, managing anxiety can become far easier.

Foods rich in tryptophan increase the amount of serotonin produced by the body, which can help people keep people calm and happy. In addition, researchers believe that a lack of serotonin can cause anxiety. Studies have found that people with anxiety disorders have far less serotonin in their blood.

A wide range of foods contain tryptophan. Bananas, nuts, and soy are all good sources of tryptophan, as are lean proteins like turkey and chicken. Tryptophan can also be found in most dairy products.

Healthy carbohydrates can also help to increase serotonin production. One of the best sources of good carbohydrates is whole grains. Whole wheat bread, brown rice, and oats can all provide an instant mood lift and a gradual reduction in anxiety symptoms.

Eat plenty of lean protein

Eat plenty of lean proteins like low-fat cuts of beef, chicken, and fish, or meat alternatives like soy, beans, and lentils. Proteins contain amino acids, which are the building blocks for cellular growth. They help us maintain the function of many systems in the body, including the skin, the organs, the immune system, and muscles.

Get your omega-3 fatty acids

They are available in fish oil supplements. Experts recommend eating fish two to three times a week or taking a supplement of about 500 milligrams a day of fish oil. Be sure that your supplement includes both DHA and EPA fatty acids. There are vegetarian versions of omega-3 supplements if you don't eat meat or fish. Omega-3 can prevent surges in anxiety hormones, mood disorders and heart problems.

Eat healthy fats

Although many of us have tried "low-fat" diets, fat is not actually our enemy. Our bodies need fats to process nutrients, to protect cells and organs, and to make hormones. What's important is what kind of fats we eat.

Consume low-fat dairy

Include low-fat dairy products in your diet. Milk, yogurt, and cheese pack in lots of nutrients. If you are suffering from loss of appetite or unwanted weight loss, dairy can provide a healthy and tasty snack. If you can't get to sleep, try a glass of warm milk before you go to bed.

Drink plenty of water

We can live for over 30 days without food, but only about 4 days without water. Drinking plenty of water can help with certain side effects of antidepressant medications, like constipation and dry mouth. It also prevents dehydration. Dehydration, even mild, can cause irritability, loss of concentration, and restlessness and contribute to anxiety.

Adults lose, on average, about 1 gallon of water every day just through respiration, perspiration, and urine. This fluid must be replaced, and the easiest way to do this is to drink water.

Eat regularly

Eat regularly throughout the day. A regular intake of calories helps to stabilize blood sugar and therefore your mood. Try not to miss any meals, especially breakfast, and have a couple of snacks throughout the day as well. Be careful, though— unregulated snacking can lead to weight gain, which will just make your anxiety or depression worse!

Consider nutritional supplements

The science is inconclusive as to whether multivitamins can play a strong role in good nutrition. However, there is no negative evidence against a basic, one-a-day type of vitamin and mineral supplement. If you decide to take a basic supplement, keep these things in mind:

- Choose a supplement with the full recommended daily intake of each vitamin and mineral. These levels are safe. However, do not take a multivitamin/mineral along with other supplements unless you are under the guidance of a medical professional.

- Let your doctor know what supplements you are taking.

- If you take a multivitamin, avoid foods that have a high vitamin A content, like liver or paté. Vitamin A is toxic at high levels.

- A multivitamin/mineral supplement is never a substitute for a healthy, balanced diet.

Set Aside Time to Worry

If you have a mild anxiety disorder, it may not dominate your life. If you have a severe one, you may not be able to leave the house, attend school, work or even shop for basic provisions. Anxiety can be truly crippling. If this sounds like you, then learn to use this tip to manage worries and fears.

Suppressing fears and worries does not always work. While you may be able to distract yourself from them for a while, they will tend to resurface later. In fact, stopping a specific thought can actually focus your attention on it and it will continue to appear in your mind repeatedly, until it has, once again, taken over.

You can take a certain time-period, such as 15 minutes a day to worry. During this time you are free to think about all of the things that worry you. But then after this time period is over, you are not allowed to spend any more of your time worrying.

Ensure You Are in A Positive Environment

The way in which we feel emotionally (and often how we act) can be profoundly influenced by those around us. Sometimes this effect is obvious and sometimes it is more subtle. We seem to actually "catch" emotions from people around us, even complete strangers. Think about that terrified stranger who sat next to you on a plane before take-off, you may not have met them before, but they'll probably send your own anxiety levels through the roof!

When it comes to people we know well and spend a lot of time with this can be even more true. Our own mental state is deeply impacted by that of other people and if you suffer from an anxiety disorder, learning to manage that impact can make a big difference in your life. Try these tips to limit your risks.

Because the impact of others can be very subtle it can help to keep a diary. Note how you feel mentally and emotionally after being around different people in your life. If you start to worry, make a note of it and try to identify what (or who) triggered the worry.

Cut back on the time you spend with individuals who make you feel down, depressed or anxious. This can be hard, depending on your relationship with the individual. Consider setting limits to what you feel able to discuss with those who are close to you, but have a negative impact on your mood.

Think about the people in your life who you trust and who you can confide in and focus on those relationships. Supportive partners, friends and relatives will help to combat anxiety disorders and their support will prove invaluable. Less supportive associates perhaps don't have your best interests at heart – you may need to assess their real motives for being around you in the first place!

Lifestyle Changes to deal with anxiety, depression, stress and chronic illness

Anxiety can cause you to feel hopeless, unimportant, out of control, and make you lose your sense of who you are. It makes you reach for comforts that are only quick fixes, and end up making you feel even worse in the end. There are many habits that you have formed in your life that could be worsening your feelings of anxiety and stress.

Limit Alcohol

Alcohol is not a terrible thing. It is normal to enjoy a couple of drinks when you are hanging out with friends or out for a celebration. It makes you feel more confident and less worried. This is because alcohol actually depresses your central nervous system. However, alcohol becomes an issue when it is used as an escape like when you find yourself reaching for a drink when you feel upset or hopeless.

Alcohol is a depressant and can make your mood worse. Furthermore, alcohol can interact negatively with your antidepressant medication, making it less effective. Alcohol also must be processed by the body and drains you of important nutrients. Several vitamin deficiencies are typical among heavy drinkers, which can in themselves lead to depression, anxiety, irritability, and aggressive behavior.

Watch your caffeine intake

Limit your consumption of caffeine. If you are prone to anxiety, caffeine can exacerbate the problem. Caffeine also contributes to insomnia, which is a common symptom of depression and anxiety. In large quantities, caffeine can also raise blood pressure and cause symptoms of depression.

Because of its diuretic effect (meaning that it removes fluid from the body), too much caffeine can cause you to become dehydrated. And it's not only coffee that has caffeine; it's tea, energy drinks, many sodas, and chocolate. If you suffer from anxiety, try to limit your coffee intake to two cups a day or less.

If you are having trouble with anxiety, consider cutting down on your caffeine intake. Coffee, and sometimes strong teas, can cause your blood pressure to increase, along with your heart rate. If you are struggling with anxiety, you most likely already feel unsettled and jittery. Caffeine can increase these feelings. Also, caffeine blocks the neurotransmitter in your brain that makes you tired, so it can affect your sleep and keep you awake.

Eat!

Anxiety can cause you to lose your appetite. However, this is dangerous because not providing your body with the nutrients it needs can worsen the way you feel. Your blood sugar decreases, and your body can get shaky and feel weak. This leads to feelings of sickness and increased feelings of panic. Always make sure that you are eating enough, even if you are having small snacks.

Lessen Social Media Scrolling

We are all guilty of it; scrolling aimlessly through social media when we have a second to spare. Social media is a wonderful tool to bring people together, but it is also a tool to make yourself feel unaccomplished and jealous. Seeing photos of other people on adventures, with their significant other and eating healthy food can make us question ourselves, "Why am

I not eating that healthy or on that extravagant vacation? I must not be as successful or healthy as that person."

Social media can eat away your day in no time. By adding up all of those times you check your phone during bathroom breaks, you have most likely spent hours on your phone. This can cause you to be upset with yourself for wasting so much time that you could have spent being productive, which will lead to more frustration with yourself and anxiety. Don't let yourself fall into this trap. It is not healthy for you and does not cultivate the growth and happiness you want to achieve.

Spend More Time with Company

Spending time with people that you love is a very healthy way to get out of your own head and feed off of their positivity. Being around people that care about you boosts your self-image and confidence. If the people that you hang out with bring you down and worsen your worries, it is time to reconsider your crowd. Good people are ones that care about you and want to be with you no matter how you feel.

Maintain a healthy weight

People who are clinically depressed often struggle with their weight, although it can be in different ways. Some people find that they lose interest in food altogether and undergo unwanted weight loss. For others, food is an emotional comfort that leads to overeating and unwanted weight gain. Antidepressant medications sometimes may affect weight, again, either in the form of unwanted loss or gain.

This seeming lack of control over your own body can just make depression worse. In addition, poor nutrition deprives your body, especially your brain, of the nutrients it needs to function in a healthy way. Unwanted weight gain often leads to succumbing to fad diets or other unhealthy eating plans. This only worsens the sense of being out of control and deepens depression, in most cases.

If you are underweight or overweight, follow the tips in this section and speak to your doctor or a nutritionist about how to maintain a healthy weight. Proper nutrition, a healthy body image, regular exercise, and good overall self-care are crucial to maintaining a good mood and remaining free of depression.

Find Something You Love to Do

Feelings of hopelessness and anxiety can rob you of your creativity and expression. As a human, it is so important to feel like you are putting your energies towards something that you are proud of. You want to feel valuable, accomplished, seen and important. Find a hobby or an extracurricular activity that you feel expresses YOUR values and YOUR interests. Paint, write, start a book club, go to the library, enter a writing contest, volunteer, start a journal...the list goes on and on. Take some time when you are meditating or having alone time to really assess your values and figure out what excites you.

Hot bath

Other activities such as taking a hot bath when getting home from work will help with anxiety. A spa or hot tub will do, too. It is a good idea to relax yourself in a hot environment when anxiety occurs. Even going to a sauna and sitting in there for about five minutes will really help with anxiety. Heating up your body reduces muscle tension that you may have and that will help decrease your anxiety. Even on cold nights, heat up a cup of hot tea, make a fire, and just sit there and relax your body and mind.

Try to get out of the house to a stress-free environment.

Go to the beach or park, bring a book with you and just sit there and try to relax your mind. Try not to think about all of the other things going on in your life. You have to take care of yourself first. Your health is very important and when you have bad anxiety this will cause other health problems. You must take the proper steps to get rid of your anxiety, it is vitally important. Go out with your friends to a stress-free environment. You have to get out of the house and be around other people every once in a while.

Sunshine on Your Shoulders

It is important to be outside. The sun provides vitamin D to your body which is essential for your health. When the sun is shining bright on your shoulders or your face, you feel more alive and active. This can help boost your mood, as the sun actually increases your levels of serotonin. The next time you are feeling down, take a step outside, face the sun, and close your eyes. Enjoy it and feel the warmth hugging your skin and let it rejuvenate you.

Being aware of your habits can give you a clearer view of what may be causing and worsening your anxiety. As soon as you can understand that the anxiety is in your own head, you understand that you have the power to stop it. Always remember to be kind to yourself. You are learning and growing in your capacity to control your mind.

Set Goals

Living with anxiety means that unknowns are looming over your head constantly. You feel as if there is always something to worry about. A deadline, an unfinished argument, work, school, everything!

Setting goals and figuring out how you can work towards them is a key way to soothing your anxieties about the unknown. When you have a plan in mind, you know exactly what you need to do and there is no opportunity to feel stuck or anxious.

Figure out what your short-term goals, slightly longer term, and lifetime goals are. What do you want to get done this week/month? What do you want to accomplish in the next six months? What do you want to achieve ten years from now? Do not limit yourself. When you have anxiety, you tend to underestimate your capabilities and your worth. Write down your biggest, most outlandish dreams and goals that you may think you are not capable of achieving. Realizing that you have goals is the first step in achieving them. It is the little steps that count the most!

This does not mean limiting yourself. This means setting your goals at a point higher than where you are at, but not so far out that you will be disappointed when you can't achieve them. You must gradually work towards your goals. For example, if you don't go to the gym at all, don't set your first goal at "Go to the gym four times a week for two hours a day." You will quickly get tired of it and find yourself discouraged.

Being very specific with your goals is necessary. If a goal is up in the air, then there is a lot of wiggle room that can lead you to stray from your path. If your goal is to improve your diet, don't just say that your goal is to "eat better every day." Something more productive would be, "Eat fruit with every meal."

If you can physically *see* your goals on paper, it gives you a lot more motivation to hold yourself accountable. Only having your goals in your head makes it simple to dismiss them and tell yourself you will start working towards them tomorrow.

Set a time frame for your goals. Do you want your diet to be fully changed in one month? If so, how can you work towards that today? There is always something that you can do today to ensure that your goals are reached, even if it is a year away. Want to have your own blog by next year? Start by writing something down today, even if it is just a topic idea for your blog. There is always something you can do.

Do not feel trapped by time and wish it would fly by so your goals can just be accomplished already. The process of working towards your goals is what makes achieving them worth it. You learn self-discipline, patience, work-ethic, and many things that are fruitful to your growth as a person and heal your anxiety. You **do have control over your life.** You

can choose what decisions you make. You **can** change your circumstances.

Your mind can trick you into feeling paralyzed and incapable of working hard and being successful. Accomplishing the goals that you set your mind to is extremely healthy for your self-confidence. Believing in yourself and seeing yourself as capable of manifesting your dreams will give you dominion over anxiety and not let it control you.

Taking Care of Your Body

There is a strong relationship between mind, emotions and body. It will be easier to relax if you know that you are taking care of your body. Try to develop healthy eating and fitness habits. Exercise and a clean diet can do wonders for your anxiety.

Also, try to sleep well and on time. If you have a healthy routine, you will have more energy to actually face and handle the ups and downs of life. Make wise food choices, develop a good sleeping habit and exercise regularly.

Talk About Your Problems with Other People

It helps if you have a trusted friend or relative who is willing to listen to your worries. Trying to contain your feelings can be very challenging. It will just allow your panic to snowball. When a person is willing to listen to your problems and vulnerabilities, you will be a bit more at ease and will realize that firstly you are not alone, and you will find that things aren't as bad as they seem.

Do not always expect that the other person will be able to comfort you completely. It is highly unlikely that the other person will be able to erase all your worries. However, talking about worries will prevent them from becoming bigger and bigger. It will prevent you from snapping at a random situation. Talking about your problems will prevent you from exploding and may assist you in maintaining perspective.

Try Connecting with Nature

There is something about the harmony of nature which is incredibly calming and relaxing. Allow yourself to be comforted by the beauty of the universe. Find solace in parks or gardens. Choose a place which will make you feel safe and grounded. If you want, you can even ask a friend to accompany you as you enjoy nature's wonders. You can also engage in a hobby involving nature. Gardening or mountain climbing is a good way to improve your relationship with the wonders around you. You'll be surprised by what a little sunshine can do in your life. You will feel lighter, better and maybe even happier.

Relaxation Breathing

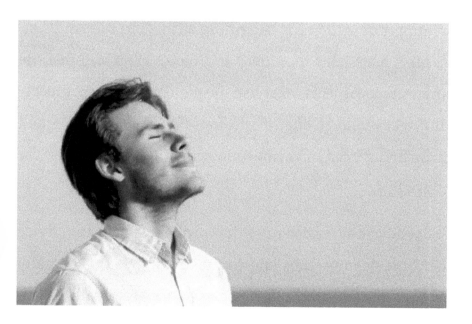

Relaxation breathing is one of the simplest methods you can apply to eliminate chronic pain. It doesn't need any training because you breathe naturally and focus on one specific thing during the exercise. Don't breathe in so fully that your muscles feel too tight or you become faint. Just take normal, comfortable, easy breaths. Do this for a maximum of five times. As you hold your breath and count, think about the position of your feet and toes.

Now breathe again through your nose, count to five and think about the position of your knees. Now breathe out through your mouth. Each time you breathe and hold, think of a different part of your body, beginning with: your toes and feet, knees, hips, arms and shoulders and hands. You will feel the calming effect of this exercise immediately. This muscle relaxing technique is one of the most popular exercise and currently being used in various medical and rehab centers for chronic pain.

Anyone who has ever been upset has probably heard the advice to take some deep breaths and count to ten, but this actually works. Breathing can be a very effective tool for dealing with anxiety. Counting breaths is one meditation method for calming anxiety that can help. It keeps your thoughts at bay because your mind is occupied with counting and thinking about your breath instead of getting stuck in anxious and negative thoughts.

You may be wondering how only breathing can relieve your pain. When you start paying attention to the way you breathe, and breathe deeply from your abdomen instead of your lungs, you can bring your anxiety levels down immediately. This is so effective that it can even calm panic attacks. It is a good idea to do breathing exercises when you are starting to feel anxiety coming on. Hold your breath by inhaling through your nose for three seconds and exhale through your mouth, then hold your breath for five seconds and exhale, again. Do this about five times in a row to lower your anxiety. If anxiety keeps occurring throughout your day, take time to do these breathing exercises. If you don't feel comfortable doing them out in the open, go to your car and do them, go to the restroom, or find a room that is empty and take the time to do these breathing exercises.

Get enough sleep

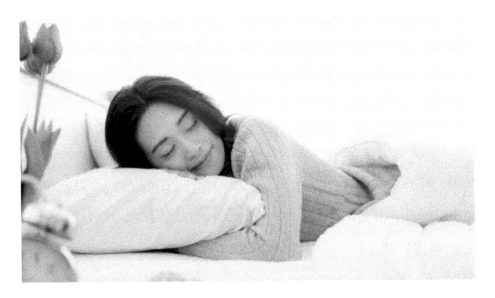

Sleep is the best medicine for everything. During sleep, the body recovers and restores. Getting sufficient sleep is very important in the process of managing pain and facilitating healing.

Experts recommend eight hours per night, though many do not get nearly that. Deep sleep and a good night's rest can be induced in various ways, with natural herbs, such as, herbal teas, warm milk, and regular exercise during the day.

Sleep is very important. It allows your brain to rest and re-charge. However, it can be difficult to sleep of you have a lot of worries on your mind. Exert conscious effort to follow a sleeping routine. Prepare your body for sleeping time. Make a concerted effort to have a beautiful rest every night so that your brain will feel more relaxed in the morning.

When you don't get good sleep, you drain your entire body and brain off essential functioning energy. In response your body and brain are reduced to anxiety, it may be hard for you to focus and make logical thoughts. On the other hand, anyone experiencing an episode of anxiety is advised to get a maximum of 8 hours uninterrupted sleep. I know I say 8 hours and it may be hard to even make yourself fall asleep. What you can do, try and prepare the environment in which you will sleep in, make it cozy, warm and secure. When you do all these things, the brain starts adjusting from anxiety mode to relief mode.

There are also various natural sleep aids on the market, and meditation techniques to get to sleep and stay in a nice deep sleep. Power naps can also do wonders during the day, 10 minutes is all it takes to revive, rejuvenate, and yes, ease the pain.

Create a Relaxing Bedroom Space

Your bedroom should only be used for sleep and intimacy, not for watching TV or checking your phone before bed. These are common mistakes that make it more difficult for your body and mind to understand that your bed is meant for sleeping. It's called conditioning. Condition your body and mind to relate to the idea that the bedroom = sleep.

For example, if you have a desk in your bedroom, it might feel like you should be working every time you go into the bedroom instead of relaxing. This can make it more difficult for you to get to sleep. If you are unable to move your work area, consider blocking it off, or disguising it in some way. Turn your bedroom into a relaxing space that allows no electronics, not even your cell phone. Pleasing décor will help also.

Create a Sleep Ritual

Sleep rituals are good for people of all ages, especially if you have trouble sleeping because of chronic pain. It helps your body and mind know when it is time for bed. This might be having a cup of herbal tea before bed, taking a hot bath, or listening to soft music. Do the same thing every night, and soon sleep will no longer elude you.

Conclusion

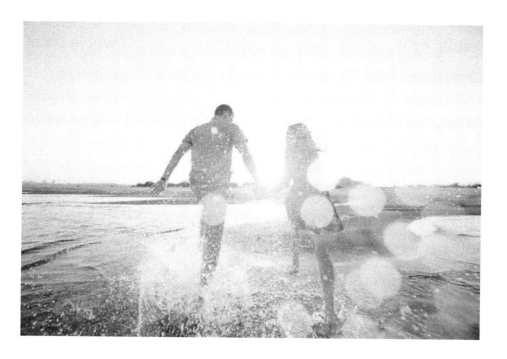

Thank you for reading this book and learning how to heal yourself. I hope you found something in this book that clicked for you; that you had the "ah ha!" moment that caused you to realize how much power you have. Anxiety and stress are tricky; they show up in daily life and have a sneaky way of making you believe that they are undefeatable. In many ways, your mind being your most powerful tool can also make it your worst enemy, but it's all about training your brain to be on your side. Remember to be patient and kind to yourself. You are learning and growing. If it's not troublesome, then it's not making any positive changes in your life. Remember that your healing process will take time, dedication, and a whole lot of faith in yourself.

Many of us know of pain as an undesirable sensation that arises from infections and injuries. However, pain is also an aftermath of certain disturbances in the normal functions of the brain and spinal cord. It can be assumed that the more stable a person's mental state is, the more he or she has the potential to tolerate pain.

More importantly, people who experience anxiety should try to get to the root of their issues. Natural remedies should be seen treatment, not a cure. People should still work to find out what the root causes of their anxiety are, and take the steps necessary to reduce the amount of stress in their lives.

All the natural remedies suggested in this book can be helpful, always know that despite what you think, there are people that want to help you, that want to see you shine and come out on top. But remember, you always have to be there for yourself, even when nobody else is. You're capable, I know you are.

References

Donna Eden, David Feinstein, Energy Medicine, 2008.

Lee Carol's channeling of Kryon at:

https://www.kryon.com/k_freeaudio.html

Lee Carol, The Recalibration of Humanity: 2013 and Beyond, 2013.

Ph.D. Mark G. Christensen (Author), D.C., M.B.A. Martin W. Kollasch (Editor), JOB ANALYSIS OF CHIROPRACTIC 2005, ISBN 1-884457-05-3, 208 p. Publisher: NATIONAL BOARD OF CHIROPRACTIC EXAMINERS

Ellen W. Cutler, Winning the War against Immune Disorders & Allergies, 1998, 582 p.

John G. Ryan, The Missing Pill, 2013

Energized for healing guided 2 minutes Meditation for good effective sleep. Video by Alexander Khomoutov at:
https://www.youtube.com/watch?v=r1b1JvGiJCM

Opening to Love – metaphysical art print for love and good luck by Elena Khomoutova at: www.lightfromart.com/node/8

Prosperity – metaphysical art print for prosperity and good luck by artist Elena Khomoutova at: www.lightfromart.com/node/12

Roses for Love – metaphysical art print for love and good luck by Alexander Khomoutov at: www.lightfromart.com/node/97

Leading-edge Healing group sessions, meditations: 16 hours audio downloads at: www.lightfromart.com/node/121

Dr. Alexander Khomoutov, Heal Yourself! Discover quantum healing energy, attract miracles and good luck in 3 easy steps, 2017.

Dr. Alexander Khomoutov, Magic of Canada: Famous Canadian Cities and Landscapes in Art Paintings, Prints and Photographs by Canadian Artists, 2017.

Abdou, A. M., Higashiguchi, S., Horie, K., Kim, M., Hatta, H., and Yokogoshi, H. (2006). Relaxation and immunity enhancement effects of γ-aminobutyric acid (GABA) administration in humans. Biofactors 26, 201–208. doi: 10.1002/biof.5520260305.

American Psychiatric Association, Diagnostic and Statistical Manual of Mental Disorders, American Psychiatric Association, Arlington, VA, USA, 5th edition, 2013.

Anderson P, Jacobs C, Rothbaum BO. Computer-supported cognitive behavioral treatment of anxiety disorders. Journal of clinical psychology. 2004 Mar;60(3):253-67.

Anderson EH, Shivakumar G. Effects of exercise and physical activity on anxiety. Frontiers in psychiatry. 2013 Apr 23;4:27.

Baek JH, Nierenberg AA, Kinrys G. Clinical applications of herbal medicines for anxiety and insomnia; targeting patients with bipolar disorder. Aust N Z J Psychiatry. 2014 Aug;48(8):705-15.

Balch PA. Prescription for herbal healing. Penguin; 2006.

Bandelow B, Seidler-Brandler U, Becker A, Wedekind D, Rüther E. Meta-analysis of randomized controlled comparisons of psychopharmacological and psychological treatments for anxiety disorders. The World Journal of Biological Psychiatry. 2007 Jan 1;8(3):175-87.

Barlow DH, Farchione TJ, Bullis JR, Gallagher MW, Murray-Latin H, Sauer-Zavala S, Bentley KH, Thompson-Hollands J, Conklin LR, Boswell JF, Ametaj A. The unified protocol for transdiagnostic treatment of emotional disorders compared with diagnosis-specific protocols for anxiety disorders: A randomized clinical trial. JAMA psychiatry. 2017 Sep 1;74(9):875-84.

Beck AT, Emery G, Greenberg RL. Anxiety disorders and phobias: A cognitive perspective. Basic Books; 2005.

Begdache L, Chaar M, Sabounchi N, Kianmehr H. Assessment of dietary factors, dietary practices and exercise on mental distress in young adults versus matured adults: A cross-sectional study. Nutritional neuroscience. 2017 Dec 12:1-1.

Clark DA, Beck AT. Cognitive therapy of anxiety disorders: Science and practice. Guilford Press; 2011 Aug 10.

de Manincor M, Bensoussan A, Smith CA, Barr K, Schweickle M, Donoghoe LL, Bourchier S, Fahey P. Individualized yoga for reducing depression and anxiety, and improving well-being: A randomized controlled trial. Depression and anxiety. 2016 Sep;33(9):816-28.

Dutheil S, Ota KT, Wohleb ES, Rasmussen K, Duman RS. High-fat diet induced anxiety and anhedonia: impact on brain homeostasis and inflammation. Neuropsychopharmacology. 2016 Jun;41(7):1874.

Garrett KM, Basmadjian G, Khan IA, Schaneberg BT, Seale TW: Extracts of kava (Piper methysticum) induce acute anxiolytic-like behavioral changes in mice. Psychopharmacology (Berl) 2003, 170:33-41.

Harvard University. What Should I Eat?: Harvard T.H.Chan School of Public Health; 2018. Available from: https://www.hsph.harvard.edu/nutritionsource/what-should-you-eat/

Hofmann SG, Wu JQ, Boettcher H. D-Cycloserine as an augmentation strategy for cognitive behavioral therapy of anxiety disorders. Biology of mood & anxiety disorders. 2013 Dec;3(1):11.

Hofmann SG, Pollack MH, Otto MW. Augmentation treatment of psychotherapy for anxiety disorders with D-cycloserine. CNS drug reviews. 2006 Sep;12(3-4):208-17.

Hofmann SG, Sawyer AT, Witt AA, Oh D. The effect of mindfulness-based therapy on anxiety and depression: A meta-analytic review. Journal of consulting and clinical psychology. 2010 Apr;78(2):169.

ESEMeD/MHEDEA 2000 Investigators, Alonso J, Angermeyer MC, Bernert S, Bruffaerts R, Brugha TS, Bryson H, de Girolamo G, de Graaf R, Demyttenaere K, Gasquet I. Prevalence of mental disorders in Europe: results from the European Study of the Epidemiology of Mental Disorders (ESEMeD) project. Acta psychiatrica scandinavica. 2004 Jun;109:21-7.

Jacobson E. Progressive relaxation: A physiological and clinical investigation of muscular states and their significance in psychology and medical practice. University of Chicago Press; 1938.

Lightning Source UK Ltd.
Milton Keynes UK
UKHW020634011220
374435UK00012B/1184